You Can Be Beautiful Beyond Breast Cancer

The strength training and diet program that changed my life post-cancer

YOU CAN BE BEAUTIFUL BEYOND BREAST CANCER

The strength training and diet program
that changed my life post-cancer

By Leslie Spencer
Foreword by fitness author Lou Schuler
Fitness Program developed by Domenick Salvatore

Meyer & Meyer Sport

You Can Be Beautiful Beyond Breast Cancer
The strength training and diet program that changed my life post-cancer
Leslie Spencer
Maidenhead: Meyer & Meyer Sport (UK) Ltd., 2012
ISBN: 978-1-84126-356-4

© 2012 by Meyer & Meyer Verlag, Aachen
Auckland, Beirut, Budapest, Cairo, Cape Town, Dubai, Indianapolis,
Kindberg, Maidenhead, Sydney, Olten, Singapore, Tehran, Toronto
Member of the World
Sport Publishers' Association (WSPA)
www.w-s-p-a.org
Printing by: B.O.S.S Druck und Medien GmbH
ISBN 978-1-84126-356-4
E-Mail: info@m-m-sports.com
www.m-m-sports.com

"Gratitude takes nothing for granted
. . . it recognizes that all is a gift from the hand of God"

Thomas Merton

There is no way I could list the names of the hundreds of friends, family, colleagues, and students to whom I am grateful. Even if your name is not listed here, it's written permanently in my heart. Here is a short list of people who made this book possible. In particular, I want to thank:

God, who has made all things work together for good in my life, even cancer.

My husband, Stuart, who demonstrated so faithfully that love is an action and not simply a feeling. Thanks for all the big and little things you did, and the ways in which you sacrificed, because you love and believe in me. I could not hope for a better partner in life.

My courageous and resilient sons, Sam and Miles.

My mom, Ruth Harrison, who loves me in a way that no one else ever could or will.

My creative, talented, and ever-faithful friend and trainer, Domenick Salvatore, who believed I was a winner from the start.

Fitness writer Lou Schuler, who took me on, out of the blue, with nothing to gain from investing in me. You told me I could write this book, and you meant it.

The competent and dedicated physicians, therapists and a great nurse who gave me such excellent medical care throughout my fight against cancer: Richard Bleicher, Joseph Delacroce, Scott Eder, Rosemary Fox, Matthew Lynch, Nenita McIntosh, Joseph Serletti, David Schaebler, Rachana Singh, Linda Smoother, Melissa Walker, and Shirnett Williamson.

TABLE OF CONTENTS

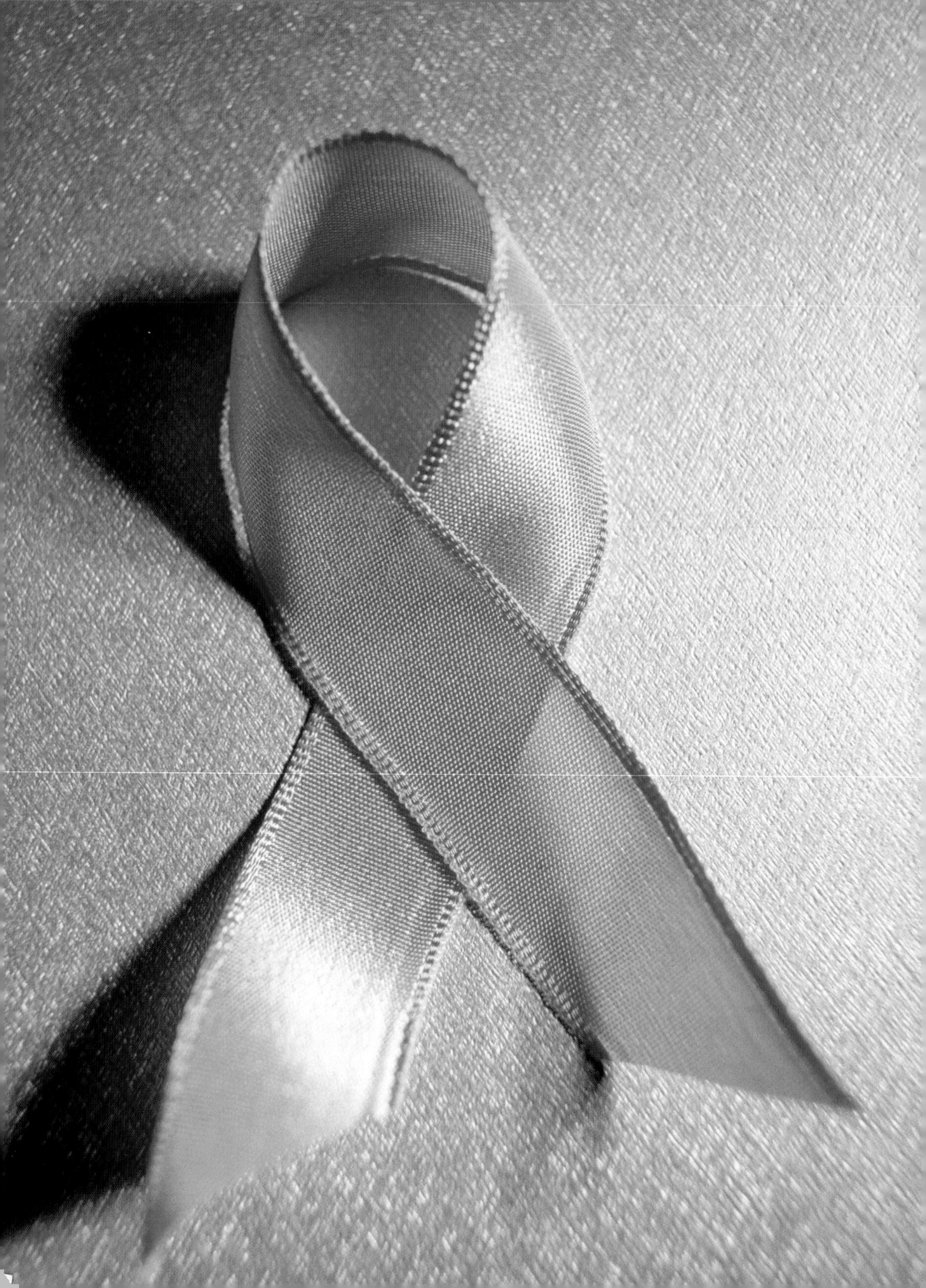

FOREWORD

by Lou Schuler,
author of *The New Rules of Lifting for Women*

FOREWORD

By Lou Schuler,
author of *The New Rules of Lifting for Women*

On December 28, 2010, I got an email titled, "Breast cancer survivor turned figure competitor appreciates your book!"

Let me be clear about one thing: My ego requires me to read that title backwards, so in my mind it said: "What a great book! By the way, I'm a cancer survivor and figure competitor."

Of course I had to open the email, and by the time I finished reading Leslie's story, I was bewildered. Why would this strong, resilient college professor take time from her day to thank me for putting a few words on paper? She said she appreciated the emphasis I put on rest and proper nutrition, especially during periods of high stress. For me, stress is a book deadline combined with driving the kids to karate. For her, it's surviving three different types of cancer, performing a demanding job, being a wife and mother, and training for a physique competition that requires a high level of muscularity combined with an almost impossibly low body-fat percentage.

And I was the one who wrote about stress and fatigue?

Since then I've gotten to know Leslie a little better, and everything new I learn is even more impressive. Most of us struggle with the simple coordination of career and family. Few of us manage to maintain a basic fitness program—much less an ambitious, competitive pursuit that forces the body to achieve a level of conditioning it actively resists—without compromising work, family, or both. And to do all that while recovering from a life-threatening illness? It seems just as impossible today as it did when Leslie first told me about it.

To call Leslie's story "inspirational" is to describe sand as "gritty." But there's a lot more here than a recitation of struggles and triumphs, as impressive as those are. Leslie's goal is to show that while recovery from cancer may dominate a person's life, it doesn't have to become one's entire life. As Leslie says, you still have choices. You can still pursue dreams, and sometimes you can even do things that wouldn't have seemed possible before you got sick.

It's a lesson that all of us, at any age or health status, can learn and apply. There will always be parts of life that are out of our control. We'll never have power over everything. But no matter how big a curve life throws at one of us, we always have options. As long as we have options, we have power over something. And as Leslie shows, a little power can go a very long way.

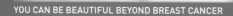

CHAPTER ONE

"You look better AFTER cancer treatment than before!"

CHAPTER ONE

"You look better AFTER treatment than before!"

Ask the average person how someone's body is likely to change over the course of cancer treatment, and they will respond with a list of symptoms that look something like this:

+ Weight loss that leaves the person looking a little too thin and weak
+ Loss of muscle mass and strength
+ A general appearance of aging skin and the lack of a healthy glow
+ Chronic fatigue, resulting in less energy for both pleasure and work
+ Hair loss from chemotherapy treatments

What you would **not** expect to hear is that this person became stronger, gained muscle, and that people told her she looked better after cancer treatment than she did before her diagnosis. Yet this is exactly what happened to me! At age 44, I was diagnosed with aggressive cancer in both breasts. In April of 2009, I began my treatment journey with a double mastectomy. In August of 2010, I celebrated its conclusion by competing in my first women's figure contest (a type of body building contest in which women are smaller and more natural looking). In between were three additional surgeries (including a hysterectomy for cervical pre-cancer), 18 weeks of chemotherapy and six weeks of radiation therapy. Of the above list of expected symptoms, I managed to avoid the first three entirely and minimize the chronic fatigue. The hair loss from chemotherapy was unavoidable, but it grew back thick and healthy-looking.

My goals in writing this book are twofold. First, I want to share my story with fellow cancer survivors to offer you inspiration and encouragement that you, too, can emerge from cancer treatment with a strong and beautiful body. Of course, every cancer survivor's experience is unique and your fitness potential during and after cancer treatment will be different than mine. But my personal experience is confirmed by some new research in exercise for cancer patients and survivors,

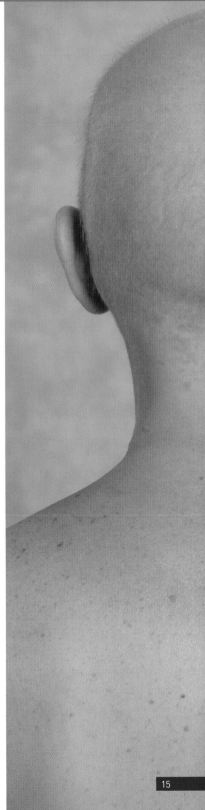

giving me the confidence to believe that you, too, have the potential to reach an improved level of fitness through your journey.

My second goal is to provide you with sound advice and a practical plan for reaching your fitness potential. As a health professional, I will provide you with trustworthy recommendations for your diet and exercise through treatment. As a cancer survivor who developed this plan by living through it, I will share my own victories and failures with you.

WHY I DID THIS
AND WHY YOU MIGHT DO IT, TOO

At this point, you may be wondering one of two questions. You may think, "Why did she do this? What made her go through all of the effort to train for and compete in a figure competition so soon after her cancer treatment?" More importantly, you may also think, "Why should I do this? Why should I put myself through the physical and mental challenge of improving my fitness level at what may be the most difficult time of my life?"

These are the perfect questions to answer at the beginning of this book because what I did (and what you can do) doesn't really matter until you know why I did it and why you might want to do it, too. I could cite some evidence about the benefits of physical activity for cancer survivors and tell you that's why I did it, but I would be lying. It's true that when cancer survivors maintain a healthy weight and fitness level, they have more positive health outcomes, sleep more

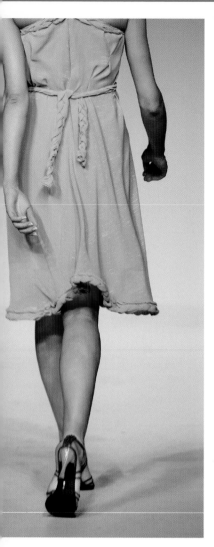

soundly, experience less stress, report greater levels of optimism and just generally fare better in life after cancer than those who don't do these things.[1] But if there's one thing I've learned in my twenty-five years as a health educator, it is that people are rarely inspired to change because they are presented with a list of facts from research studies. They may believe it and think it's a good idea, but they probably won't act on it until they have a personal passion for it. Factual information leads to "head knowledge," but it takes something else to cultivate an "understanding of the heart," which is what you need to really grab onto an idea and live it.

So are you ready to hear the real reason why I persevered through cancer treatment to train and compete in a figure competition at its completion? It's this: I did it to experience victory over cancer in a direct, unexpected, and powerful way. I wanted to be known as the woman who was training for an athletic competition through her cancer treatment, not just a woman who was going through cancer treatment. Was cancer the dominant theme in my life during that time? Of course it was; I would be in a state of denial if I said otherwise. But that didn't mean that cancer was the *only* theme in my life. Resilient people are able, even in the toughest situations, to identify options and make choices. They feel empowered instead of powerless. Now, it's vitally important that I balance this by saying that none of us has complete control in life, and that we are not all capable of the same achievements. Part of my resiliency was to recognize when some of my strategies weren't working and to be willing to change my tactics and expectations. I'll share my weaknesses and limitations with you as freely as I share my successes as I tell my story. Paradoxically, I found that when I acknowledged and accepted my weaknesses, it made me stronger. False pride is flimsy and easily undone, while genuine humility is much tougher than it appears on the surface.

I also found it highly encouraging to have a vision for something to look forward to and be excited about beyond cancer. I spent a lot of time on the sofa in the weeks after each surgery and chemotherapy treatment. Daydreaming about how I would look and feel on stage, after all of the treatment was over, carried me through some rough days. Searching the internet for a posing suit, watching videos to learn the stage walk and figuring out the details, such as how to get the best spray tan (a requisite for figure competitors on stage), kept me occupied with a project that was important to me and *didn't have anything to do with cancer*. When you have cancer, it's easy to fill every day with medical appointments and research on your treatment options and decisions you have to make. I remember taking "days off" from cancer, i.e., days in which I would have no cancer-related appointments, phone calls or internet research. Planning for the figure competition was a very satisfying way to spend a day off from cancer.

Finally, you might be wondering why I chose to pursue a figure competition and not a triathlon or other fitness goal. The answer is that the figure competition gave me something unique that a different goal would not have provided in the same way. It allowed me to feel beautiful to the point of being stage-worthy in a "glitter" bikini and four-inch heels! After having both a mastectomy and hysterectomy, it was special to me to feel beautiful, feminine, and sexy after losing the parts of my body that are associated with being female. Competing in a triathlon would have given me a sense of victory, but not the same affirmation of my femininity and beauty.

MY POSING SUIT ARRIVED IN THE MAIL TWO MONTHS BEFORE THE COMPETITION. I MODELED IT IN MY HOME WHEN I RECEIVED IT.

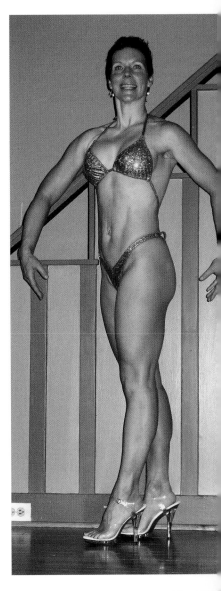

WHY ME?

It's the classic cancer question – "*why did this happen to me?*" Many people have asked me if I struggled with this, especially since I lived such a clean and healthful life prior to cancer. There is no history of breast cancer in my family, and the genetic tests I took showed that I don't carry the genes for it, either. You might be surprised, but this is not a question that has bothered me. I don't say this as a point of pride, but simply out of honesty. I have been blessed with an ability to make peace with my cancer.

With that said, I do have some thoughts on the "why me?" question. The first one is that I got off easy. When I consider my whole life, the benefits I have enjoyed far outweigh the hardships. I have a great marriage to a wonderful and supportive husband, two terrific sons, and a large, extended family that surrounds me with love and care. I have an excellent education and plenty of resources, unlike the majority of the world's people, to live a full and fulfilling life. And when I just consider my cancer treatment alone, the benefits increase. I had a network of over 200 people around the world (including a group of African pastors) who prayed for me consistently for a year. My employer allowed me to take an extended, paid medical leave, so my job and finances were not a worry. I have a great health insurance plan and access to some of the finest cancer care in the country. Friends and neighbors cleaned our house, walked our dog, entertained our children and cooked us more meals than we could eat. Now, *there's* a reason to ask "why me?" Why did I deserve to have all of these good things happen to me? We seldom ask that question. Perhaps it's part of our culture of entitlement, to believe that we are owed an easy life where we always get what we want. I had to face this and say "why not me?" when considering why I developed cancer. If I am going to accept all of the blessings in my life, then maybe I also need to accept the challenges.

I also found that living through cancer treatment brought about some very positive experiences and opportunities I would not have had without first having cancer. My pursuit of figure training is more meaningful as a result of cancer. I also made a great connection and am working on a research project with Dr. Kathryn Schmitz, a University of Pennsylvania researcher who has pioneered research on

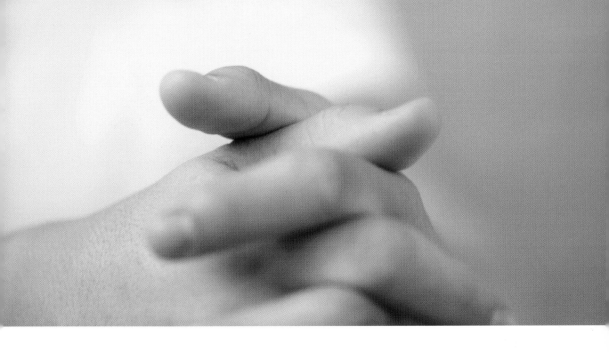

the benefits of strength training for breast cancer survivors. I wrote this book because cancer has given me a story to tell and a passion to tell it!

My intention is not to trivialize my, or anyone's, cancer. I am well aware that my chances of having cancer again are higher than the average person, and I know that I may die from cancer someday. I have also met many cancer survivors who have a prognosis that is not as good as mine and who live with much more hardship than I do. Yet, I am reminded of Dr. Paul Brand's classic book, *Pain: The Gift Nobody Wants*.[2] Dr. Brand was a physician who specialized in leprosy treatment among the poor in India. He made a critical discovery in the 1950s, when he realized that the major problem faced by those with leprosy was an inability to feel pain, which prevented them from avoiding injury. They would experience serious bodily harm because they had lost the natural protective mechanism triggered by pain, such as pulling your hand away from a hot stove. I think we've lost an appreciation of this in the United States. We spend our lives trying to avoid pain and stay comfortable, sometimes at all costs, but it is pain that provides a vital corrective mechanism to move us away from danger and into live-giving habits and attitudes. Cancer, and cancer treatment, is physically and emotionally painful, but it has allowed me to understand and experience some

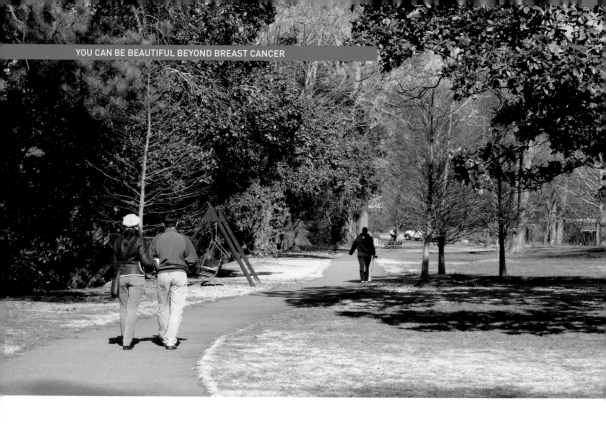

very important things that I would have missed had my life remained easy and unchallenged.

You might be surprised to hear that there were elements of my treatment that I enjoyed and even miss, now that I am back to my normal life. One thing I miss is the time that cancer treatment afforded me. For eight months, I had the freedom of putting my career and other obligations on hold. It was all I could do to care for myself physically and maintain relationships with my family. Even though I often didn't feel good, I still enjoyed long, quiet walks in my neighborhood and lots of time to read and reflect on my thoughts. I loved the solitude it afforded me, which I rarely experience in my normal life. I still try to create these quiet moments, but they are not as leisurely and unburdened as they were during my treatment, when I could easily give myself permission to be still and quiet.

HOW MY CANCER AFFECTED MY FAMILY

"Mom, how often do people die from the kind of surgery you're having tomorrow?" My 11-year-old son posed this question to me the night before my hysterectomy, which was my third surgery. This brave boy witnessed the aftermath of two breast surgeries and the effects of chemotherapy and radiation therapy on his mother with few to no comments about the experience. I naively thought he was handling it without too much anxiety, but his question showed me that there was much more he was thinking than expressing in words. From the start, my husband, Stuart, and I spoke openly and comfortably at home about my diagnosis and the treatment to come. We were thoughtful about the level of detail we shared in front of our sons (the younger one was six), but we believed the experience would be even more frightening if our boys suspected us of keeping secrets from them or perceived that they were not 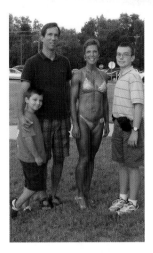 allowed to talk about it. Prior to each surgery or treatment, we provided a basic explanation to them and then allowed them to ask as many or as few questions as they wanted. Overall, I think this strategy was successful, but, in hindsight, we would have encouraged our older son to participate in a support group offered by a local hospital for kids who have a parent going through cancer treatment. His performance in school was academically strong, but he withdrew from his friendships during the year I was going through treatment. His teachers told us that he ate his lunch and spent recess alone, preferring to read a book rather than join the other kids. While the teachers frequently invited him to talk to them or be part of the group, they were sensitive to his wishes and gave him the space he wanted. About four months into my treatment, Stuart and I felt that it would be good for him to have something new and positive in his life, and he joined the Boy Scouts of America. He connected well with his leader and the other boys, and became less isolated as he fit into this social circle. We were grateful to see this happen.

At age six, our younger son did not appreciate the deeper implications of my cancer and treatment. All he knew was that his mom was now available *every day* to play board games and make jigsaw puzzles! How could he not be excited about that? To him, my disease meant the steady delivery of meals and treats to our house, long visits from his grandparents, and lots of play dates with his friends at their homes. He thought it was all pretty fun, from what we could tell. He was curious

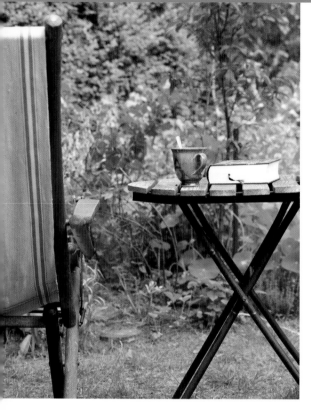

about my bandages and surgical drain tubes, but they were more a source of fascination than anxiety. As he grows older, we will be very interested to hear what his perceptions are of that time in our family life, and perhaps then we will know if we wished we had handled him differently.

One question I'm frequently asked is how my sons felt about having their mother don a bikini and four-inch heels to parade across a stage, flexing her muscles for the crowd. I think I'm safe in assuming that most of us would have a hard time picturing our own mothers doing that! For my older son, the figure competition became a project for us to share together. He loves technology and gadgets, so it was a natural fit for him to become my webmaster as I launched my first blog (my sister-in-law created my second, and current, blog). He was also my photographer and videographer, documenting the final months of my training, a short video I made in which I tell my story, and the competition itself. He loved this role, and I think it helped him find a positive focus out of the otherwise negative experience of having his mom undergo cancer treatment. He didn't seem to mind my revealing stage costume too much, but then he had a job to do (video-recording) during my time on stage and a reason to be proud of the photos and footage that were then posted on my blog.

True to his outgoing, spotlight-loving personality and age, my younger son loved the flashiness of the crystal-studded pink bikini, and he gave no thought to me wearing it publicly. In fact, I think the whole experience seemed normal to him (doesn't everyone's mother do this sort of thing?). In the year following the competition, he has shown a lot of interest in weight training and eating a "clean" (i.e., lean and healthful) diet himself. He decided to give up his beloved chicken nuggets after learning that bodybuilders don't eat that sort of food, and he now has me "train" him with some light hand weights so his muscles will get stronger.

SURGERY, CHEMOTHERAPY, COMMITMENT, AND SEX

There are a number of ways in which Stuart and I don't fit the stereotypical roles of husband and wife, despite our traditional family structure and life. He's a much better and more creative cook than I am. I handle all of our finances and investments, and he's happy to not be bothered with it. He has more friends than I have, including several very close male friends with whom he shares his more intimate thoughts. And of the two of us, he tends to be more sensitive to the emotional climate of our home and marriage. Sometimes he can more accurately pinpoint what I'm thinking or feeling about a situation than I can! As we navigated my cancer treatment, he brought the gift of awareness – of himself, of me and of our relationship – to our situation, so I asked him what he would say if he were writing this paragraph. He responded that adversity has a way of either driving people apart or bringing them closer, and that we have a more intimate bond because our shared vulnerability brought us closer to each other. He was reminded of our wedding vows, especially the part where we promised to stay together "in sickness and in health," and of the powerful influence of strong role models in his family and our church; other men who supported their wives through cancer treatment and other major illnesses.

Stuart once heard that divorce is the end result for two-thirds of the couples in which the wife undergoes breast cancer treatment, and that one of the reasons for the deterioration of the relationship was the loss of sexual interest from one or both partners. Either the husband stopped finding his wife attractive, or the wife stopped believing that she was desirable, even if her husband felt otherwise. I know of one breast cancer survivor who has given up dating after being rejected by a potential mate who could not accept the fact that one of her breasts was slightly misshapen due to a lumpectomy. Of course there are boyfriends and husbands out there who do *not* feel this way (mine is one of them), but breast cancer surgery and treatment have an impact on sexual self-perceptions and relationships, even very healthy ones. It's beyond the scope of my story to uncover all of these issues, let alone respond to them, but I would at least like to share the experience that Stuart and I have had in this aspect of our relationship.

Much to my surprise, Stuart and I enjoyed sexual intimacy throughout my treatment. The fact that I had scars on my chest where breasts used to be and that I was bald did not keep either of us from wanting to have sex. At first, I

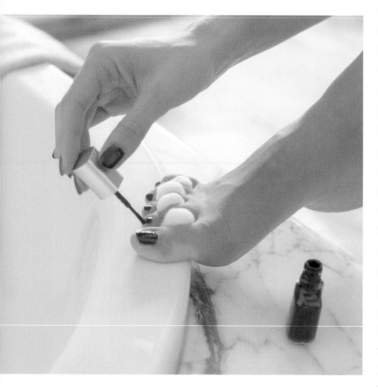

would cover my head with a scarf and wear a tank top, but over time, we got used to how I looked and neither of us felt a need to do that. I focused on feeling attractive in other parts of my body; for example, I wore make-up every day and gave myself weekly pedicures. Cancer treatment heightened my desire to feel attractive and sexy in the ways that I could, and I enjoyed pampering myself. I learned that cancer treatment is like running a marathon, not a sprint. Through the long duration, there are more difficult periods and there are easier periods. Enjoying sex during the easier periods was an unexpected pleasure; it felt good to us both physically and emotionally.

Since my breast reconstruction has been finished and my health and lifestyle have settled into a new version of "normal," Stuart and I continue to enjoy sex, although it's a little different now and may always be that way. One thing that's changed is that my energy level, although pretty high compared to most people my age, is not what it used to be. I get tired faster and run out of energy for lots

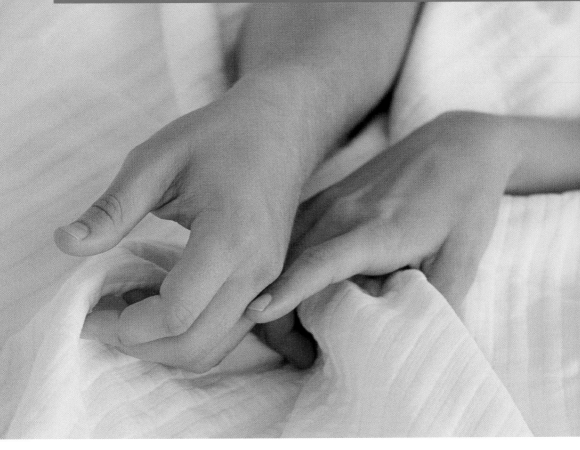

of things, including sex sometimes. Of course, this comes with aging, whether you've had cancer or not. Any middle-aged, working professional with kids will tell you, if they are honest, that they are sometimes too tired for sex. But cancer seems to have accelerated the pace of this experience for me. A second change is that my reconstructed breasts (with silicone implants) look very nice and natural, but they don't feel natural. They are uninvitingly firm to the touch for my husband, and to me, they feel mostly numb when they are touched. For couples for whom the woman's breasts were a significant part of their sexual pleasure, there might be some disappointment in reconstructed breasts. It's been relatively easy for us to enjoy other aspects of sex and touch apart from my breasts, though.

I've heard people say that what makes you sexy is simply your belief that you are, in fact, a sexy and desirable person. It has less to do with what your body looks like and more to do with your attitude about yourself, your partner and the experience and meaning of sex. Cancer has taught me the truth of this.

REFERENCES

1   There is strong evidence to support the claim that exercise is good for cancer patients and survivors. A few reputable summary sources that are concise and reader-friendly include:

+   National Cancer Institute. (2010). Guidelines Urge Exercise for Cancer Patients, Survivors. *National Cancer Institute Bulletin, 7 (13)*.

+   American Cancer Society. *Physical Activity and the Cancer Patient,* Accessed March 14, 2011 on www.cancer.org.

+   Komen, S. G. *Facts for Life: Physical Activity.* Accessed March 4, 2011 on www. komen.org.

2   Yancey, P. and Brand, P. (1993). *Pain, The Gift Nobody Wants*. Michigan: Zondervan Publishers.

"YOU LOOK BETTER AFTER CANCER TREATMENT THAN BEFORE!"

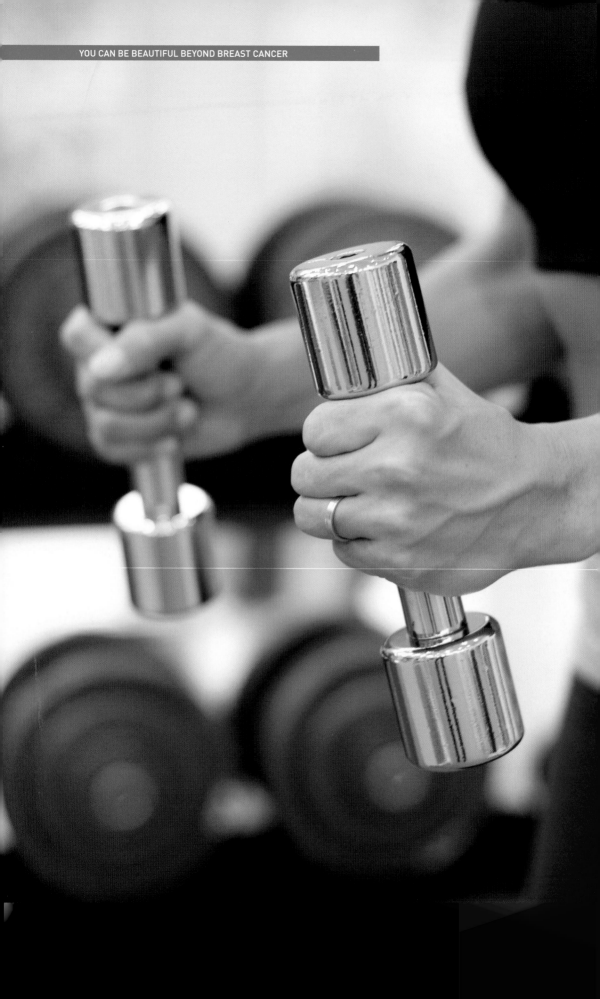

CHAPTER TWO

"You'll never lift more than 10 pounds again!"

CHAPTER 2

"You'll never lift more than 10 pounds again"

I was a month into my cancer treatment, coping with all of its demands and surprises, when I discovered a potentially big hole in my plan to become a competitive figure contestant. I wasn't supposed to lift anything heavier than ten pounds – ever. My first thought was "no way, this can't be right!" Further

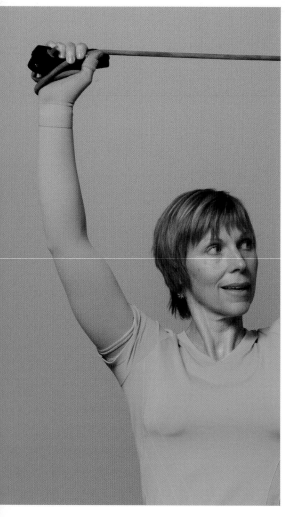

investigation on several reputable websites confirmed that this was, in fact, a common recommendation to breast cancer survivors who have had lymph nodes removed from the armpit area. Most of these sources exhibited what I now call "Old School Thinking" and it goes like this: Breast cancer surgery with lymph node removal increases your risk of lymphedema, an accumulation of fluid, in your arms and hands. This is exacerbated by lifting heavy objects. What was the proposed solution? Don't ever lift a heavy object again for the rest of your life, including your groceries, your golf clubs, or your grandchild.

Now, lymphedema is not a condition to take lightly. In fact, lymphedema can be a greater source of anxiety than the loss of a breast for some cancer survivors, particularly if the swelling it causes is severe. When a woman has lymph nodes removed from the armpit area, her body has more difficulty keeping fluid circulating and not accumulating in her

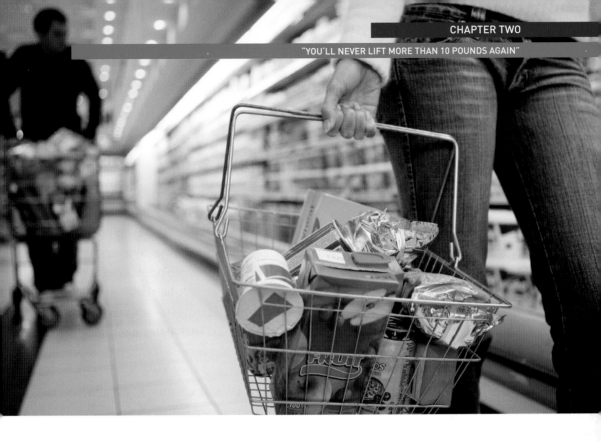

arms and hands. Certain triggers, such as a sudden force or pressure on the arm, can lead to dramatic and permanent swelling. Yes, I said permanent. Once you have lymphedema, it doesn't go away. You can keep it from getting worse if you are vigilant in treating it, but you will always have it.

I have slight lymphedema in my right arm, which is about one centimeter larger than my left arm because of the swelling. I also have some numbness in the skin of my right armpit, which is another common symptom. The good news is that I've managed to weight train with very heavy weights (sometimes holding up to a 50-pound dumbbell in each hand) without having the lymphedema become worse, but I have built up to this amount of weight carefully, and I always wear a compression garment on each arm and hand every single time I exercise.

SAFE, BUT DEFINITELY SORRY

By following the Old School Thinking pattern, breast cancer survivors can minimize their chances of having lymphedema, but at a very high price in their quality of life. By avoiding lifting anything more than 10 pounds, these women shortchange themselves in many ways. Research shows that, without regular exercise, breast cancer survivors are more likely to gain weight, feel anxious, feel tired more often, lose their ability to do many of the activities of daily life and generally miss out on things they used to enjoy.[1-2]

With disappointment, I began to doubt whether it was wise of me to pursue my figure training goal given the information I was reading about the potential risks of weightlifting for cancer survivors. For better or worse, I am driven toward achieving my goals and this news wasn't enough to convince me that I couldn't become a figure contestant, yet I also try to be smart and realistic about my goals. So I began the task of digging deeper into the underlying evidence for this "no lifting" admonition for breast cancer survivors, and what I found surprised me.

Very few research studies on the prevention of lymphedema after breast cancer surgery examined the impact of exercise at all, and those that did began with the assumption that certain forms of exercise could only worsen the condition. What was really frustrating was that, up until very recently, no research had ever been conducted (or at least made public) to assess the value of weight training for breast cancer survivors, the drawbacks of *not* engaging in weight training, and whether there could be a better solution to this problem. Certainly in my case, this weightlifting restriction would end my dream of becoming a figure contestant.

ENTER OUR HEROINE, DR. KATHRYN SCHMITZ!

I remember the day I first discovered an article on the work of Dr. Kathryn Schmitz, a researcher from the School of Medicine at the University of Pennsylvania, who has devoted her professional life to improving the physical fitness of breast cancer survivors. Finding a description of her study on weight training for breast cancer survivors who've had lymph nodes removed was like seeing the rays of the sun breaking through the clouds after days of rain. Her research provided answers to my questions and allayed my fears, and I was once again hopeful that I could realize my dream of becoming a figure contestant. I call her Katie now, as she's become both a friend and colleague with whom I have the privilege of working.

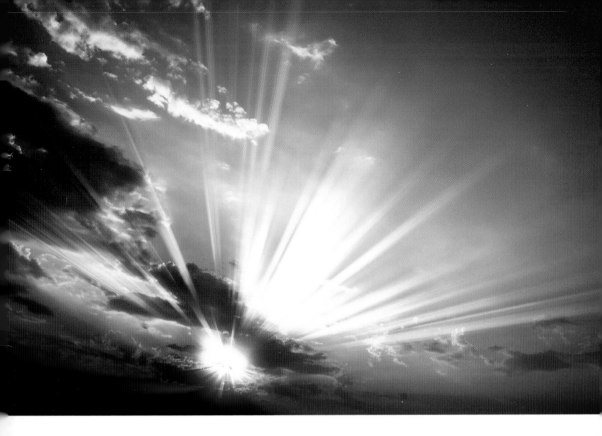

THE SURPRISING EVIDENCE
THAT OVERTURNED THE "OLD SCHOOL THINKING"

In 2005, Katie began recruiting breast cancer survivors into what would become the largest and most scientifically rigorous of any research study on the effects of weight training on women after having breast surgery and/or chemotherapy and radiation treatment. The study is called PAL, which is short for Physical Activity and Lymphedema, and the results have been impressive enough to be published in both the Journal of the American Medical Association[3] and the New England Journal of Medicine[4].

All of the women in the PAL study had surgery to remove lymph nodes; 141 of the women had lymphedema at the start, and 154 of the women did not have lymphedema, but were at risk of developing it. These two groups were further divided; half were randomly assigned to participate in an upper-body weight training program two times a week and the other half did not do any weight training. (The random assignment is important here. It helps to ensure that the results of the study were due to the training program and not for some other reason.) Guess which groups of women showed less anxiety, less fatigue, more strength,

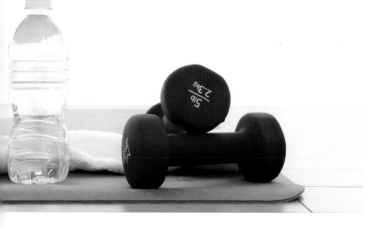

improved self-image, and, most significant, *less lymphedema* at the end of a year? If you guessed the women who participated in weight training, you're right! For the group of women who didn't have lymphedema at the start, only 11% of those in the weight training group (as compared to 17% in the non-training group) showed any lymphedema a year later. For the women who had lymphedema at the start, those who engaged in weight training had fewer complications, experienced less anxiety about their lymphedema, and were physically stronger than those who did not train with weights when they were assessed a year later. We know that lymphedema won't go away once you have it; what's important here is that upper-body weight training did not cause additional swelling and that the weight-training women felt more confident in themselves and their ability to manage their condition, compared to the non-weight-training women.

An unlikely meeting through *Philadelphia Inquirer* columnist Art Carey

A staff writer for the *Philadelphia Inquirer*, Art Carey produces a weekly column on health and fitness topics. At the risk of making him sound old (he's not), Art is a Philadelphia institution with a loyal readership that has followed him for decades. His impact is far-reaching, and this book is a case in point. If it had not been for Art's column on Katie Schmitz and her work, I would not have known about her and would not have written to him with my story. In a subsequent column, Art told my story and mentioned in it that Katie's work was instrumental in my decision to pursue figure training. Well, Katie read the column about me and contacted me. In the months that followed, we met and became both friends and working colleagues, and we have Art to thank for it.

TRAINING "SMART" AFTER BREAST SURGERY

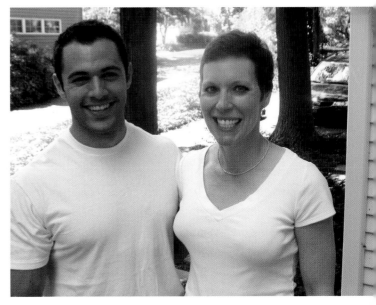

LESLIE WITH DOMENICK, HER TRAINER

At this point, I want to make a few important points before you start hefting any dumbbells. First, every PAL participant who had lymphedema wore compression sleeves on her arms and gauntlets on her hands for each exercise session. If you have had lymph nodes removed and/or radiation to one or both armpit areas, you need to know what these are. The sleeve covers your arm from shoulder to wrist, and the gauntlet is like a glove without fingers; both gently compress your limb to keep it from swelling. You also need to have a set and wear them without fail every time you exercise or exert pressure on your affected arm(s), *even if you have not shown any signs of lymphedema*. Since I had lymph nodes removed from both armpit areas, I wear sleeves and gauntlets for both arms and hands, even though I only have lymphedema in my right arm. I put them on *each and every time I exercise without exception*. I also wear them when I rake leaves, help move heavy furniture or fly in an airplane. In short, if pressure will be exerted on my arms by any activity or situation, the sleeves and gauntlets go on first. Compression garments aren't cheap, and you can do more harm than good if you don't wear a set for which you have been measured and fitted, so please don't wear someone else's sleeves or wrap your arms in bandages as a substitute. Ask your breast surgeon for a recommendation to a physical therapist who specializes in treating breast cancer patients (many don't) and have the therapist fit you for a set of sleeves. You also need to know that they wear out; I replace mine every six months. My health insurance covers about 90% of the cost, for which I am grateful, and it's worth finding out what your insurance will cover.

Second, the PAL participants worked with fitness trainers who received special training to work with cancer patients and survivors. For this study, Katie partnered with several branches of the YMCA in her area and provided instruction to the staff who would be guiding the PAL participants through their weight training sessions. Please do not assume that your average personal trainer knows the specific needs of a client undergoing breast cancer treatment. Unless the trainer has been specifically educated to work with cancer patients and survivors, she or he is probably not a good choice for you. Nationally, the YMCA has taken a lead in providing programs for cancer survivors and is a good place to start when you are looking for a fitness center to join and/or a personal trainer. The LIVESTRONG program at the Y provides qualified fitness trainers and instructors to work with people going through cancer treatment, and I recommend it to women who are currently in or have recently completed breast cancer treatment. Not all YMCA branches have instructors trained to work with breast cancer survivors, though, so ask specifically if your instructor has this training.

My trainer is Domenick Salvatore, and he designed the fitness program featured at the end of this book. In a neat twist of fate, Domenick transitioned from being my student to being my teacher. As a graduate of the health promotion and fitness management major at Rowan University, he was my student for four years. In the last semester of his senior year, I asked him to train me in our fitness laboratory, as I thought he was a particularly talented trainer. It was during that semester

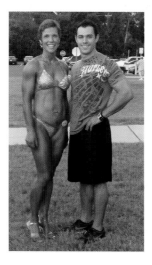

that I was diagnosed with cancer. Domenick partnered with me through all of my treatment, and as I prepared for the figure competition, studying the specific needs of cancer patients and survivors and tailoring the training program to my changing physical condition and ability. After graduation, Domenick earned the Certified Strength and Conditioning Specialist (CSCS) credential from the National Strength and Conditioning Association, which is one of the most respected personal training certifications available. Domenick now works for Katie as a research assistant, applying his fitness knowledge in new studies of exercise for women at high risk for breast cancer.

STILL NOT CONVINCED? THERE'S MORE EVIDENCE

Some of you who know a thing or two about research may be saying at this point "yes, that's great, but these are the results of just one study. It takes more than one research study to establish exercise guidelines we can trust." Fortunately for you, Katie did her homework and participated in an effort to find and analyze all of the published research on exercise for breast cancer survivors. While the PAL study provides the strongest and best evidence, she and her colleagues found an additional 32 studies examining the effect of exercise in general (including, but not limited to, weight training) on breast cancer survivors after they had completed treatment and 22 studies examining the effect of general exercise on women during chemotherapy and radiation treatments.[5] To make sure that their conclusions were trustworthy, they only included well-designed, experimental studies that met criteria acceptable to most researchers. Here's what they found:

+   *All* of the studies examining safety showed that it was safe for women to exercise, both during and after treatment,
+   *All* of the studies examining changes in strength, flexibility and the ability to perform tasks of daily living showed improvement,
+   Half or more of the studies examining changes in body weight, aerobic fitness, anxiety levels, fatigue and body image showed increases in these areas, and
+   *Seven* studies specifically documented the benefits of upper-body weight training after breast cancer treatment without causing or worsening lymphedema in the participants.

HOW COULD SO MANY PHYSICIANS BE SO WRONG FOR SO LONG?

Chances are likely that you, as a cancer patient, have found a surgeon, a medical oncologist, and a radiation oncologist whom you trust and like. These physicians are probably competent and caring, and they are working hard to give you the best treatment available. Chances are equally *unlikely*, though, that they are familiar with the newer research on weight training for breast cancer patients and survivors. They will either omit discussing exercise with you at all, or they will simply encourage you to do cardiovascular exercise, such as walking or jogging, and give you a warning to be careful about lifting anything heavy. As recently as ten years ago, they probably would have specifically discouraged you from exercising during your treatment.

Why? Why would otherwise smart and skilled physicians fail to give their patients good advice on a topic so critical to the patients' quality of life and long-term health? This would make a great discussion topic, as I'm sure there are many possible answers to this question. So, at this point, I humbly offer my opinion on this matter. Let me begin by stating that, without exception, I have a great respect and appreciation for the many physicians who have cared for me throughout my treatment. They have been everything a patient wants in a good physician, and they were all supportive of my goal to train for a figure competition when I told them about it. Yet, none of them broached the topic of exercise with me, nor did they ask me if I had compression sleeves when I told them I was training with weights. Perhaps they sensed that I was knowledgeable about exercise and didn't need their direction, but I don't think this was the reason. I think their lack of advice to me on this topic was due more to the fact that exercise was not within their realm of expertise and/or that they assumed my other physicians were discussing it with me. I've heard this combination of factors called the "silo effect," where each physician operates within his or her narrow specialty (as if he or she was in a silo) and it's up to the patient to coordinate the different recommendations from each physician, as well as fill in the gaps that none of them are addressing. I'm not finding fault with them, though. The volume of information related to their specialty alone is overwhelming; keeping up with it is daunting enough, much less becoming an expert on something new. Most have also received little or no training to assist patients in changing their lifestyles by improving their diets or adding exercise, and they (like most of us) prefer to stick to what they know they can do well. Combine these factors with the pressure from managed care to maintain a heavy patient load, and it's not a surprise that many good physicians aren't finding the time to study this information.

The conclusion I've come to is that, with breast cancer treatment (and probably treatment for other conditions, too) you need to advocate for yourself and view

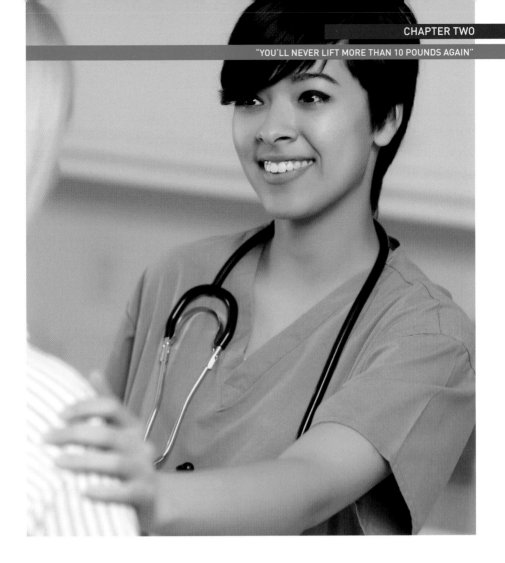

yourself as a partner in your care. I always shared what I was doing with my physicians and sought their input, but I did not rely on them to tell me everything I needed to know.

FINAL THOUGHTS FROM KATIE AND HER TEAM

In 2010, Katie and her research team published a great piece in the journal produced by the American College of Sports Medicine, in which they explain to fitness professionals how to best understand and serve clients with cancer.[6] Much of what they said in this article is instructive for those of us who are cancer survivors, and I'd like to summarize their ideas here, with a few comments of my own.

Do what you can and don't worry about what you can't do. On many days after surgery or a chemotherapy treatment, the most I could do was to walk to the end of my driveway and back to the house. As someone who could run several miles without stopping prior to cancer, this did not feel like much of an achievement. Still, I got up and did the best I could do, knowing that I would eventually regain my strength and stamina. Remember that there is a benefit to getting up and moving whenever and wherever you can as you move through treatment, even if it seems like an insignificant accomplishment at the time.

Be flexible in your expectations of yourself. As I moved through treatment, my training program and goals changed on a weekly (and sometimes daily) basis. I would have become very frustrated if I had not been willing to change my expectations of what I could achieve on a given day, based on how I was feeling and how my body was responding. You will have days when you feel energetic and others when you feel sick or tired; adjust your expectations to match your ability each day.

You may experience some treatment effects years after treatment is over. The professionals call these "persistent effects" and I can tell you first-hand that they are real. For years after cancer treatment has finished, you may experience episodes of fatigue, digestive problems, hormonal changes and their resulting symptoms (such as hot flashes), and/or a loss of bone density, to name a few of the more common persistent effects. In later chapters of this book, I'll tell you more about the fatigue and irritable bowel syndrome that have affected me post-treatment. For now, I'll simply tell you that these long-term effects have had an impact on my fitness training, and I have had to make allowances for them. You should be prepared to do the same.

Plan to educate your fitness trainer about your treatment, symptoms and needs. Don't assume that your trainer will know how you feel or what you need, even if she or he is experienced in working with cancer patients. Your symptoms and challenges will be different from those of other women who've had breast cancer.

So that's the evidence behind the plan. In the following chapters, I'll share the fitness and nutrition plan with you and, hopefully, inspire you to try it for yourself!

REFERENCES

1   Schmitz, K. H., Troxel, A. B., Cheville, A., Grant, L. L., Bryan, C. J., Gross, C. R., Lytle, L. A., Ahmed, R. L. (2009). Physical Activity and Lymphedema (the PAL Trial): Assessing the safety of progressive strength training in breast cancer survivors. *Contemporary Clinical Trials, 30*, 233-245.

2   Speck, R. M., Gross, C. R., Hormes J. M., Ahmed, R. L., Lytle, L. A., Hwang, W. T., Schmitz, K. H. (2010). Changes in the body image and relationship scale following a one-year strength training trial for breast cancer survivors with or at risk for lymphedema. *Breast Cancer Research and Treatment, 121* (2), 421-430.

3   Schmitz, K. H., Ahmed, R. L., Troxel, A. B., Cheville, A., Grant, L. L., Smith, R., Bryan, C. J., Williams-Smith, C. T., Chittams, J. (2010). Weight lifting for women at risk for breast-cancer related lymphedema: A randomized trial. *Journal of the American Medical Association, 304* (24).

4   Schmitz, K. H., Ahmed, R. L., Troxel, A. B., Cheville, A., Smith, R., Grant, L. L., Bryan, C. J., Williams-Smith, C. T., Greene, Q. P. (2009). Weight lifting in women with breast cancer related lymphedema. *New England Journal of Medicine, 361*, 664-73.

5   Speck, R. M., Courneya, M. S., Masse, L. C., Duval, S., Schmitz, K. H. (2010). An update in controlled physical activity trials in cancer survivors: A systematic review and meta analysis. *Journal of Cancer Survivorship, 4* (2), 87-100.

6   Schmitz, K. H., Courneya, K. S., Matthews, C., et al. (2010). American College of Sports Medicine Roundtable on exercise guidelines for cancer survivors. *Medicine and Science in Sports and Exercise, 42* (7), 1409-1426.

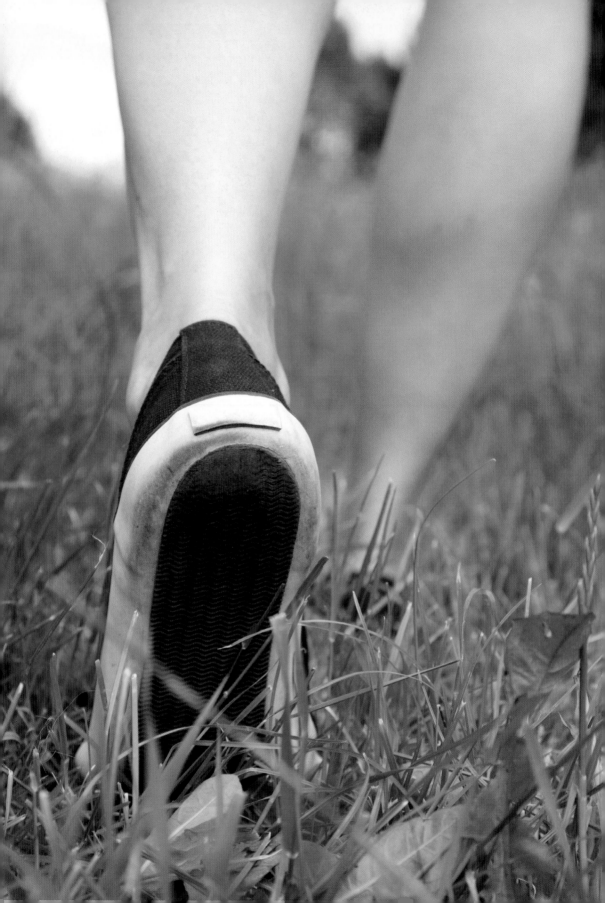

CHAPTER THREE

My exercise goal today is walking to the mailbox

CHAPTER 3

"My exercise goal today is walking to the mailbox"

Now that you know the thinking behind the plan, it's time to get specific about the plan itself. How did I train through cancer treatment? In this chapter, I'll explain my approach to fitness training in detail so that you can follow it, too. Specifically, I will show you how I rehabilitated my body during the six weeks after each surgery, how I exercised through the ups and downs of six cycles of chemotherapy, my method for regaining my upper-body range of motion and maintaining it through radiation therapy, and how I progressed to a demanding training regimen for figure competition preparation once my body was ready for it.

I USED TO WORK OUT, NOW I TRAIN

So far, I haven't differentiated between the terms *training* and *working out*, but it's time to do that. When I talk about the way I exercise, I am intentional in my

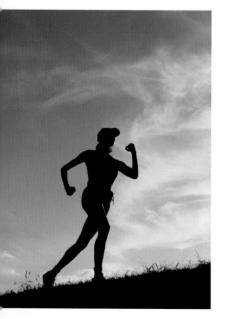

use of the word *training* as opposed to *working out*. I owe my enlightenment to fitness author Lou Schuler, who says that *training* is what you are doing when you have a goal in mind, such as bigger, stronger muscles; weight loss; or an athletic competition. *Working out* is what happens when you exercise without a plan for progress.

Before I had cancer, I was only *working out*. Exercising made me feel better and helped me keep my weight under control, but I put little thought into what I was doing or why. I focused primarily on running and using the elliptical trainer in the gym. My resistance training was sporadic and, I now realize, largely ineffective. It's different for me now and much more motivating, as you'll see in the rest of this chapter.

"TRAINING" POST-MASTECTOMY

I have to use the word training loosely in describing what I did in the five weeks following my double mastectomy. Of my four surgeries, this was the most difficult from which to recover and it required the most determination through which to rehabilitate. It was an amputation of a sizeable part of my body and, although my natural breasts were not that big, I felt a difference in my balance initially. I had immediate reconstruction, with tissue expanders placed under my chest muscles at the time of the mastectomy. It would take another 10 months for them to be expanded out to the size of my permanent implants, and I had a completely flat chest for the first two months.

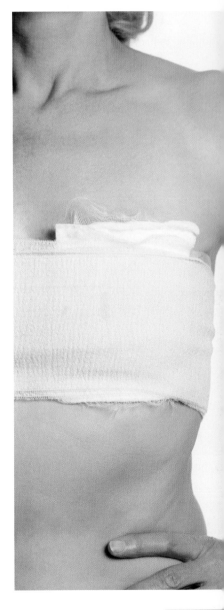

At this point, I must note an important caveat. There are different types of reconstructive breast surgery. Instead of silicone or saline implants, many women have a procedure known as a TRAM flap, in which fat and muscle from the abdomen are pulled up into the chest to form breasts. This is an even harder surgery than the one I had, as it involves both the chest and the abdomen and requires a longer recovery time. If you have had a TRAM procedure, your post-surgical recommendations may be more limiting than were mine. The evidence is strong in support of moving back into a fitness program after a TRAM procedure, but the timeline may be different than for someone like me having tissue expanders and implants. Please discuss your post-TRAM fitness plan with your surgeon and allow more time for recovery if you need it.

I endured a week of moderate to severe pain after my mastectomy, during which I counted the minutes until I could legitimately take my next dose of Percocet. I'll

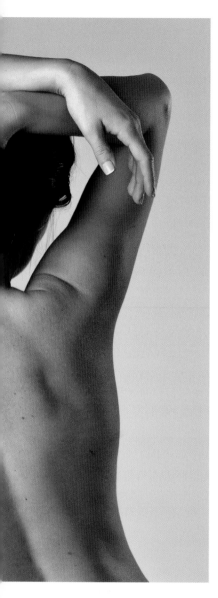

admit I cheated and took them early a few times when the pain was unbearable. Still, I made it my goal each day to stand up for a few minutes every hour and raise my arms over my head. At the hospital, I stood up the day after my mastectomy and the nurse taught me to "walk my fingers up the wall" to regain the ability to raise my arms above my head. I've heard that when women don't do this right away, they often find that they cannot raise their arms above their shoulders once they do try to lift them.

My guiding rules for activity after surgery were to pay close attention to how I felt and to follow the instructions of my surgeons. Feelings of pain, weakness, light-headedness and discouragement were all signs to me to sit or lie down and rest. When I felt good, though, I would walk around the house and in our yard throughout the day, raising my arms over my head every few hours. Using deep breathing and meditation exercises helped me fight post-surgical grogginess, delay my need for pain medicine, and feel better.

During the next five weeks, I progressed to increasingly longer walks until I was walking for a mile in my neighborhood three times a day. I paid attention to my body's signals and stopped walking if I felt pain, weakness or dizziness, and I set a pace that allowed me to walk without discomfort. I stretched daily, adding more exercises as the weeks progressed. In the second week, I added simple, standing leg exercises. With my hand on the wall for balance, I did standing leg lifts, knee lifts, leg curls and squats. It was too soon to move in a way that caused me to engage my chest muscles, though, so I didn't. I always stopped before I felt pain or discomfort. By the third week, I began sitting on a stability (exercise) ball instead of a chair for periods of time. I was very careful to position the ball in

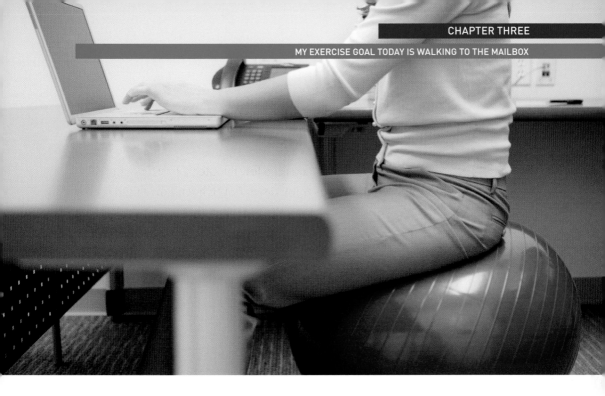

a place where I could support it and be confident that I wouldn't accidentally roll off the ball, but this is not as hard as it sounds. This was a way to slightly begin engaging the core muscles in my abdomen, lower back and hips. I could also shift position on the ball and do slight "hold and squeeze" exercises for my rear end and thighs, which felt good and alleviated the numb feeling I got from sitting in a chair all day. You may not be able to do this so soon after a TRAM flap.

By the fifth week, I was feeling much like my "old" self. I was free of pain, energetic, and doing all the activities of daily living. The pace of my three mile-long walks became brisk, and I also performed a total body stretching routine once each day. During the fifth week, with my surgeon's clearance, I started doing a few upper-body exercises holding a 5 lb. weight. Unfortunately, my progress was halted by an unexpected development.

At the end of the fifth week, I was back in the hospital for a second surgery. It turned out there was cancer in my right breast, too, that hadn't been detected in my mammogram. I thank God that I had the foresight to have the right breast removed anyway, as it was the post-mastectomy biopsy that revealed this second cancer. My surgeon hadn't removed any lymph nodes from my right armpit during the mastectomy, as we didn't think there was a reason to do so. This time around, he removed eleven lymph nodes from my right side. There was also a need to

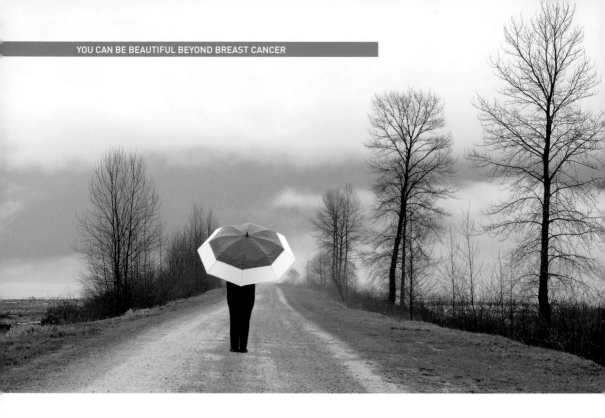

remove ten additional nodes from my left side, as the first surgery yielded only two and one of them was positive for cancer. After having lymph nodes removed from both armpit areas in this second surgery, I once again began the rehabilitation "training" program of standing, stretching and slowly walking as I regained my strength and my body healed.

THE EMOTIONAL DRAIN OF SURGICAL DRAINS

I never knew what a surgical drain was until I had my mastectomy. When I awoke from my surgery and surveyed the scene of my bandaged chest, I saw them for the first time. They were clear, plastic bulbs, each about the size of a tennis ball, with tubing that led directly into my body. Yes, there were four little holes in my skin, two on each side of my chest, through which the plastic tubes entered, draining off excess fluid from the surgical site. Held in place by surgical stitches, they wiggled and *pinched* whenever I touched them or moved in a certain way. They were to become the bane of my existence for the next three weeks until they were removed. Honestly, living with surgical drains was perhaps the hardest part of the whole treatment process for me. I was aware of them during every waking moment and thought, at times, that I would go crazy trying not to be irritated by them. After my second surgery, I had two more drains in my chest, and after my third surgery, I had one drain in my abdomen.

My post-surgical fitness program had to be tailored around the drains. I found that tying a piece of ribbon around my torso, over the tubing, helped reduce the movement of the drains by holding them still and keeping them close to my body. If it had not been for this, I probably could not have walked much due to the movement of the drains and subsequent pain it caused where they entered my body. Anchoring the drains to my torso also enabled me to do more stretching without fear of causing them to move.

The presence of surgical drains may make you hesitant to move very much until they are removed. Of course, you don't want to do any movement that could dislodge the drain and your surgeon will give you specific instructions to prevent that from happening, but there is plenty that you *can* do, including walking, stretching and the simple post-surgery leg exercises, such as standing knee lifts, leg curls and calf raises. This is one of those moments where you need to decide that you *will* do the exercises, despite your fears and your inclination to curl up in a ball and channel surf until the drains are gone. Starting to walk was the hardest part when I had drains. Once I was moving, though, I felt better. I also learned how to hold my arms and how to walk in a way that didn't bother the drains, and the exercise itself improved my mood and spirits. Try it; I think you'll find that it's not as hard as you imagine it will be.

TRAINING WITH LYMPHEDEMA

As I noted in the previous chapter, I have lymphedema in my right arm. It came upon me suddenly and dramatically one day when I was training my upper body with kettlebells (a type of hand-held weight) about four months after my mastectomy. I remember clearly how it happened. Standing in the family room with a kettlebell in each hand, I was performing an overhead shoulder press. In the middle of the second set, my right arm began to visibly swell (about a one centimeter increase), and I felt tingling in my hand and fingers. My instincts told me to put down the kettlebells, raise my right arm above my head and gently

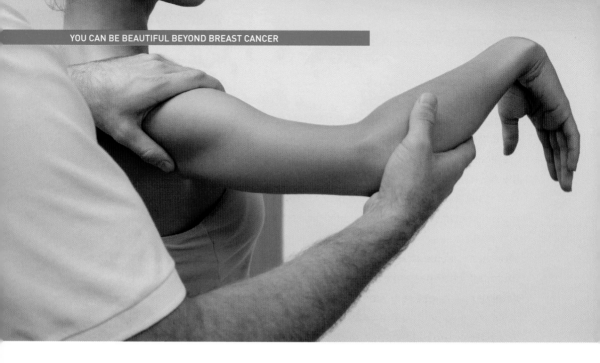

massage it with my left arm in an effort to bring down the swelling. It turns out that was the right thing to do, although I was massaging my right arm with too much pressure, I later learned from Linda, my physical therapist. I had been seeing Linda already to help increase the range of motion in my arms, so she was the first person I contacted when the swelling began. In one of those early visits, Linda had told me about the value of wearing compression sleeves and hand gauntlets during exercise. I was planning to get a pair, but obviously, I didn't plan to get them soon enough! She measured me for the garments and now I wear them without fail every time I exercise. Through her treatment, plus a daily self-massage using a technique she taught me to do at home and wearing the compression sleeves each time I exercise, I have been able to reduce the swelling of my right arm considerably and keep it from getting worse, even though I now lift very heavy weights. The lymphedema will never go away entirely, but I can keep it to a minimum by following some good guidelines.

First, I wear the compression garments on both arms, even though my right arm is the only one with lymphedema. Since I had lymph nodes removed on both sides, both arms are at risk. Second, I wear them every single time I exercise, including running, brisk walking or doing leg exercises. It's not just direct exercise involving the arms that can trigger lymphedema; any vigorous activity that raises your heart rate can cause this swelling. Third, I gradually built up to lifting heavy weights. Someone who has not had lymph nodes removed can probably progress faster to heavier weights than I did, but that's o.k. I train very intensely, but I started at lower weights and gradually increased the amount to protect my arms. Finally, I replace my garments every six months, since I wear mine six days a week and they lose their compression capability over time. I am fortunate to have a good health insurance plan that covers almost all of the cost, and it's worth finding out if your insurance will cover the cost for you.

One bit of advice I will give you is to ask your surgeon to refer to you a physical therapist who specializes in treating lymphedema soon after your surgery, if you have lymph nodes removed. Have the therapist work with you to increase your range of motion and measure you for compression garments. Don't wait until you have a problem to ask to see a physical therapist and don't assume your surgeon will recommend it without you specifically asking for it. As wonderful as my physicians have been, none of them recommended physical therapy or compression garments, but when I asked for a referral, they were more than happy to give me one.

TRAINING THROUGH CHEMOTHERAPY

My chemotherapy treatments were tough. Many women with breast cancer will have eight treatments every two weeks and alternate between drugs. I had six treatments, but I received all three standard drugs (Taxotere, Adriamycin and Cytoxan) at every treatment. My treatments were three weeks apart for this reason. It would take until day 11 post-treatment for me to feel somewhat normal again, so I would have a little more than a week of feeling strong before the next treatment began.

My treatments were on Monday afternoons and lasted 4 1/2 hours. My worst day was the first Thursday after a treatment, so I had a massage on that day from a massage therapist who was specifically trained to work with cancer patients. The massage on my worst day helped me get through it more easily.

Each day without exception, I would make myself get out of bed, get dressed and take at least one slow walk in my neighborhood. It was hard to get out of bed, but once I was out, I would start to feel better. I would also do a 20-minute stretching routine each day. As the days went by, I could walk and stretch a little more until I reached the eighth day, when I would add in some resistance training. By day 14, I could jog two miles and do a fairly intense resistance training workout, which I would do each day for the week prior to my next treatment. I am convinced that this made me stronger for the next chemo treatment, and my chemotherapy symptoms were reduced because of my training.

Every Monday morning Domenick came to my house to work with me. Even if it was day eight and I couldn't do much, he came anyway and I did as much as I was able. Psychologically, this was very important to me. It helped me feel less like a cancer patient and more like a healthy athlete. How I perceived myself was critical to my ability to stay active. The great thing about training all through chemotherapy is that I was able to maintain my fitness level so that, at the end of cancer treatment, I was still in good physical condition and ready to prepare for body building.

HOW CANCER CHANGED THE WAY I TRAIN

Quality instead of quantity

I've always been an overachiever at school, work, volunteer activities and, well, just about everything in my life, including exercise. When I was pregnant with my first son, I taught a group exercise class a week before my due date and participated in a class on my due date. He cooperated by waiting five more days to come into the world.

For better or worse, this trait extends to my figure training. Like many American women, I fear weight gain and the loss of my fit physique, and I was driven to do intense, long workouts six days a week. I took my rest day begrudgingly, knowing that it was good for me but wishing I didn't need it. You are right to think this sounds obsessive, although I hate to admit it. As a healthy woman prior to cancer, I was able to do this without injury or discomfort. After cancer it was a different story.

One thing I wasn't prepared for were the symptoms I experienced after I completed my cancer treatment. Sure, I knew what would happen to me during treatment; I expected to be tired and lose my appetite after chemotherapy and have the pain and discomfort that comes with recovery from surgery. What I didn't expect was to have new symptoms develop a year or more after I finished treatment. In my case, there were two major ones. The irritable bowel syndrome I developed led to changes in my diet, and I'll talk more about that in the next chapter. The episodes of chronic fatigue, lasting a week or more at a time, challenged my attitudes and beliefs about training and changed the way I approached it, and that's what I'll discuss here.

You might be surprised to learn that I did not have bouts of fatigue as I was going through treatment. Although I had to carefully rehabilitate my body after each surgery and chemo treatment, I would work my way back to long, intense, frequent training sessions. My body seemed to adapt well enough to this approach – I had no lingering injuries, and I felt good most of the time. It wasn't until after I competed in my first figure competition and was into my second year post-treatment that fatigue enveloped me in a way I had never experienced before. From a discussion with my physical therapist, also a cancer survivor, and some online reading, I have learned that post-treatment fatigue is common among cancer patients, and that I may have episodes of cancer-related fatigue for the next several years.

I was halfway through the fall semester, working hard at school and home, training hard and pushing myself almost every waking hour of the day, when my body began to revolt against the expectations I was placing on it. My daily dose of Tamoxifen, a common chemotherapy drug taken by breast cancer survivors for five years after treatment, was suppressing estrogen production in my body. The ensuing hot flashes woke me up in the middle of the night and kept me from falling back to sleep, intensifying the effect of my demanding daily routine. I had to do something I had never done before. I took a week off of work because of debilitating fatigue. A physical exam confirmed that I didn't have the flu, a fever, the Epstein Barr virus or mononucleosis. I was simply exhausted from pushing too hard for too long. It was hard to accept this change in my body and its abilities, and I fought it at first. As my energy level began to increase, I made myself get right back to my training program. As you can imagine, this led to a lapse into exhaustion and the cycle repeated itself for about eight weeks, until I finally started to wise up and change my fundamental beliefs and approach toward training. I experienced what could be considered a paradigm shift; it was like taking off an old pair of outdated glasses and putting on a new pair. Until I started seeing my old training strategy through the new lenses, I didn't realize the degree to which I was misguided in pushing myself into counterproductive training sessions.

In short, I learned that quality matters more than quantity when it comes to reaching my training goals. Lou Schuler makes this point so clearly in his New Rules of Lifting book series. He says that it is during the rest periods in between workouts that your muscles become bigger and stronger, not during the training itself. I knew this before, but I don't think I truly appreciated it, especially for my own body. Lou provides a great discussion of the importance of rest – between sets in a workout, between workouts, and for a week at a time between training programs. In other words, resting is just as important as training to gain muscle strength and size.

My body knows what it needs (and doesn't need)

So how do I do it differently? First, I stop and assess myself before I train. I pay attention to my energy level and enthusiasm for the training session. Am I looking forward to it? Do I feel like I can give it my all and have a productive session? If not, then I don't exercise that day. Now, some of you are thinking, "Well, if I only exercised on days when I *really* wanted to, I would never do it!" My response is that you probably don't obsess about training and have difficulty resting. You very well *may* need to push yourself a bit to overcome inertia, despite having the physical energy to have a good training session. But for someone like me who struggles to rest even when my body is crying out for a break, answering these questions is a good self-test in deciding whether or not to train. Second, I limit my resistance training to five days a week (and sometimes three or four if I don't pass the self-test questions). My goal is to work as hard as I can during training, aiming for steady and consistent improvements from one session to the next.

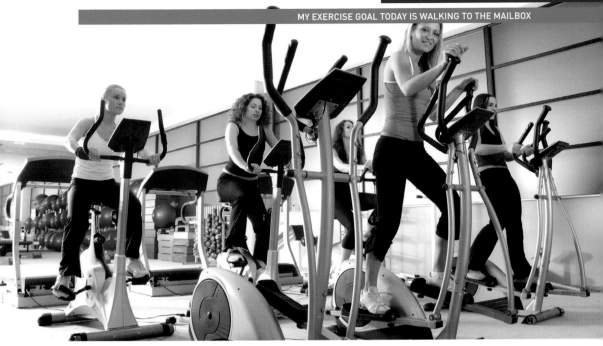

Third, I stop the training session when I reach the point where I am not performing at my best. I've made resistance training my priority, with cardiovascular training secondary, given my goal to compete in figure competitions. This means that I am willing to skip the cardiovascular component at the end of the workout if the resistance training part has used all of my energy.

THE DREADED BIG, BULKY MUSCLES

Spend some time in the cardio section of any gym and listen to what many women have to say about weight training as they relentlessly work the treadmill or elliptical trainer. They will likely tell you that, yes, a little weight training would be good for them, but what they really care about is burning fat (hence the hour-long sessions of cardiovascular work) and they are afraid of developing *big, bulky muscles*. In their view, having noticeable muscles is worse than having excess fat (which they can't seem to get rid of, despite years of walking, biking, group exercise or using the elliptical trainer). If this is one of your fears, let me set you straight before you read further, because I am most certainly recommending that you lift *heavy weights* (heavy for you, that is, at your current strength level) and try your very hardest to get bigger muscles. I want to frame this around two reality checks.

Reality Check One: It takes years of disciplined, demanding, daily training to get big muscles.

In fact, most female figure contestants would find it laughable, if not slightly offensive, to hear an undeveloped woman express her fear of getting big muscles. No one gets bigger muscles by accident; you have to really WANT them to get them. Even then, you will be limited by genetics and your physiology as to how big your muscles will get.

Reality Check Two: As you age, you either get bigger muscles or you get fatter.

There's no other option. Many women have a vague notion of wanting to look toned without having bigger muscles. They don't understand two important things. First, only teenage girls have the ability to look firm and smooth without growing their muscles. Forty-something women can't have that body again. Second, when you see an adult woman, especially one over age 35, with what you would call good muscle tone, you are probably describing a woman who lifts heavy weights and has bigger muscles as a result.

Two factors conspire together to make women fatter as they age. Estrogen reduction is one major culprit. As you near menopause and then enter it, you will begin a decade of making less and less estrogen. If you are a breast cancer survivor and your cancer was estrogen sensitive, you have the added disadvantage of taking drugs, such as Tamoxifan or an aromatase inhibitor, to suppress estrogen production in your body. You also must avoid supplements and foods, such as black cohash or soy, which stimulate estrogen production. Of course, hormone replacement therapy is completely out, although few women are interested in it these days because of the other associated health risks. You may even have had a complete hysterectomy (like I did) or oophorectomy, in which just the ovaries are removed, to stop ovarian estrogen production (your adrenal glands, fat tissue and skin will continue to produce some estrogen). A second contributor to fat gain as women age is the slowing of your metabolic rate, or the rate at which your body uses calories. Starting at age 30, your body's metabolism slows down by about

100 calories per week *each year*.[1] In other words, every year of your life after age 30, you need to make up for an additional 100 calories per week by exercising more and eating less. (Notice I said "and," not "or"; I believe both strategies are necessary to prevent fat gain.)

Building bigger muscles is the best antidote. Weight training will help you increase your muscle size and strength and reduce body fat. The mere presence of more muscle in your body will require that it use more calories to maintain those muscles, even when you are not exercising.

Prior to weight training, I spent years on the elliptical trainer, stair climber and jogging in my neighborhood. Rarely was I complimented on my body. As I started weight training and building bigger muscles, I began hearing a steady stream of compliments, including that I looked buff, young for my age, and just generally better than I had for years. Perhaps someone is secretly thinking that I look to "bulky," but I doubt it. My husband tells me (and sometimes he tells other people) that he thinks I look hot! I don't need any more confirmation than that to keep training.

WILL HEAVY TRAINING HURT THE BREAST IMPLANTS?

My implants are comfortable, but I always know they are there. I am particularly aware of them when I am training my chest muscles, since the implants sit *underneath* those muscles, which have been stretched to accommodate them and hold them in place. When I bench press a heavy load, I can feel the strain of my chest muscles against my implants and a little voice in the back of my mind asks "will the implants rupture? Will they dislodge?" The answer to these questions is a confident "no," according to Dr. Joseph Serletti, Chief of Plastic Surgery at the Hospital of the University of Pennsylvania. Dr. Serletti also happens to be my surgeon and observes the impact of my training program on my implants at my regular physical exams. According to Dr. Serletti, as long as you are careful not to exert your chest muscles during the six weeks after surgery, the implants won't be harmed by exercise, including upper-body weight lifting with heavy weights.

While I have not been able to find any published information on the impact of post-mastectomy breast implants on fitness training, I believe it's a logical deduction that the presence of breast implants has changed the anatomy and physiology of my chest. I have adjusted my training program to accommodate it. The primary adjustments I've made are to increase the amount and frequency of the shoulder joint rotation exercises I do and to focus on training the muscles in my shoulders, upper back and chest to be strong and flexible in order to avoid injuries.

Domenick created a series of exercises that we present in the Appendix to build both strength and flexibility in the chest and shoulders, help you rehabilitate after surgery, through chemotherapy and radiation therapy, and prepare your body to follow a weight training regimen to achieve your fitness goals. We encourage you to make the commitment now to try the program and experience the positive results in how you look and feel!

REFERENCES

1   McArdle, W. D., Katch, F. I., Katch, V. L. (2008). *Sports and Exercise Nutrition,* (3rd edition). Philedelphia, PA: Lipincott Williams and Wilkins.

Note: On p. 462 of this text, the authors describe evidence that supports the recommendation to increase weekly exercise by 1.4 miles beginning at age 30 to counterbalance the slowing down of metabolism due to age. I calculated that the additional 1.4 miles would burn approximately 100 calories in a 150-pound person, which is the basis of my recommendation in this chapter of my book.

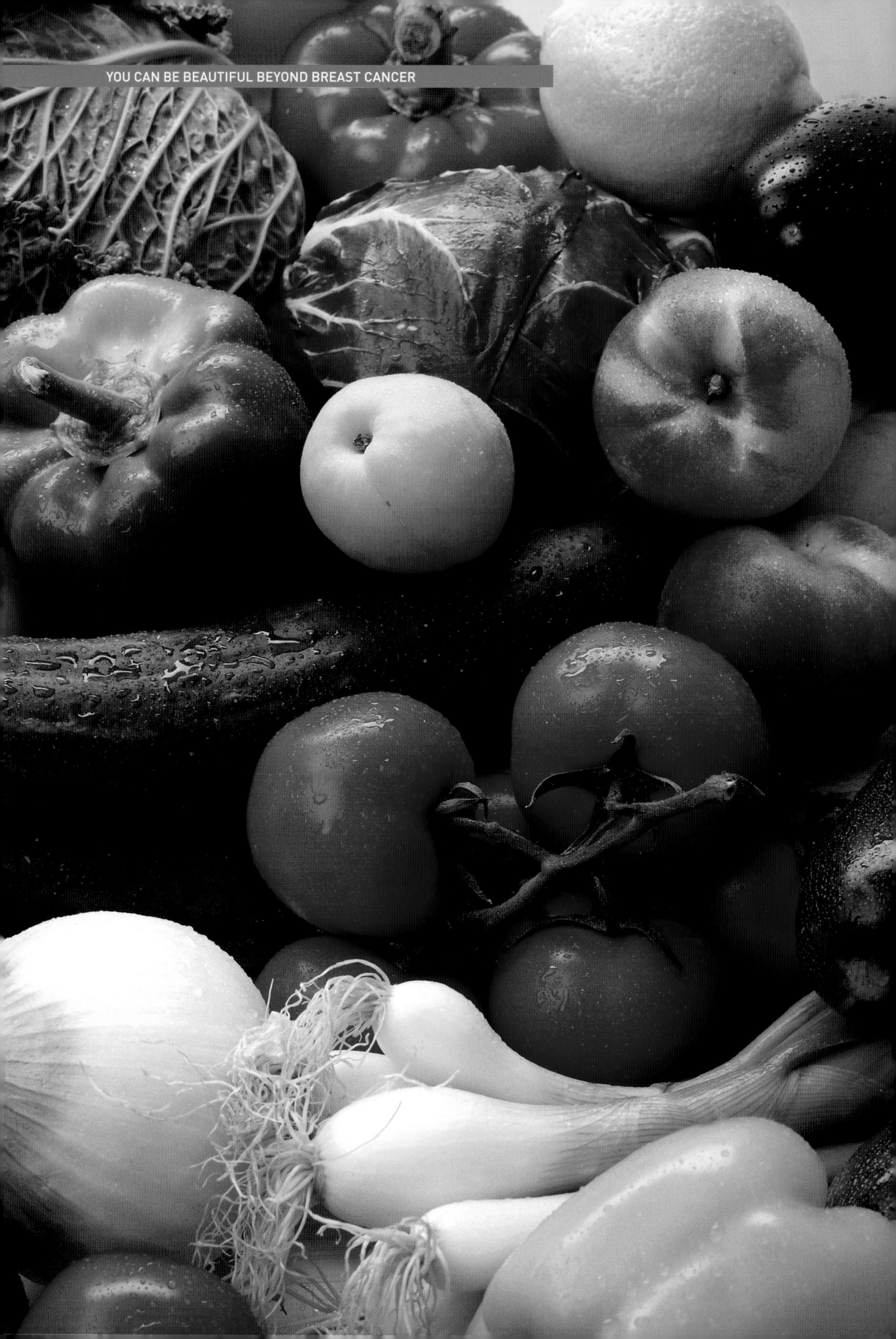

CHAPTER FOUR

Everything tastes like dirty pennies

CHAPTER 4

Everything tastes like dirty pennies

You'll face different kinds of nutrition challenges as you move through surgery, chemotherapy and radiation. Not only did my appetite vary from wanting no food to eating constantly, I also found that many foods tasted worse to me during chemotherapy in particular. I regained most of my sense of taste after chemotherapy ended, but it didn't return completely. Now I find that flavors need to be stronger for me to taste and appreciate them. Milk chocolate has lost its appeal; only dark chocolate will satisfy me! Cancer treatment permanently changed how foods taste and what I can digest without discomfort.

My goal in this chapter is to provide you with good advice and guidelines for each of these phases of treatment, based on both my professional knowledge and my personal experience. I'll also describe the particularly challenging diet of a figure contestant, including the pitfalls and dangerous practices followed by some, and tell you how I navigated that component of my preparation safely and effectively.

Nutrition 101: A quick review of the basic ideas

In this chapter and the next, I refer to a number of nutritional concepts, such as the percentages of calories that come from carbohydrates versus protein and the problem of a ketogenic diet. Some readers may appreciate a review of the basics before reading the rest of the chapter, so here it is.

What is a calorie?

One of my favorite moments in the movie *Super Size Me* was when Morgan Spurlock interviewed people on the street, asking them "what is a calorie?" While everyone he asked was extremely familiar with the term, no one could quite explain what it was! We know we're supposed to not eat too many of them, and that some foods contain a lot of calories, while others contain few calories, but most

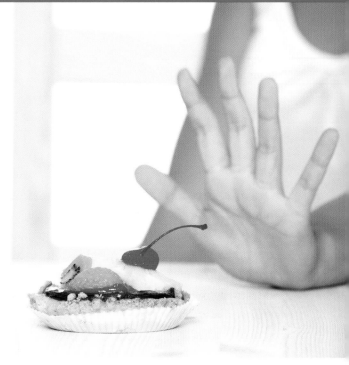

of us can't really tell you what a calorie is. Let me provide you with a simple definition. A calorie is a unit of measure we use to determine the amount of energy that one serving of a food gives us. In nutrition, the words "calorie" and "energy" mean the same thing; just like gasoline provides energy for your car to run, calories provide energy for your body to function.

The six major types of nutrients and why each is important

I'm a fan of simple, practical definitions, so here's another one. A nutrient is something you eat that is good for your body in some way. Of the 40 plus individual nutrients that we know about, we can categorize them into six different groups.

Carbohydrates are found in all of the food groups. We generally divide them into complex carbohydrates, such as the starch in potatoes and bread, and simple sugars, which include things like table sugar, the fructose found in fruits and the lactose in milk. They have one job in the body, providing us with energy, and they do this job very well. You need carbohydrates to be healthy and have the energy to exercise. Whole grains, like brown rice and wheat bread, are better choices than white rice and white bread. Vegetables and fruits are also great sources of carbohydrates.

Fats have been highly underrated in recent years. They are also a source of energy for the body, but they do other important jobs, like transport certain vitamins to your muscles and organs. Fats from plant sources are better for your heart than animal fats, as they help keep your cholesterol levels down. Vegetable oils in small amounts and the natural fat found in avocados and nuts are where you'll find the plant-based fats.

Protein is found in both animal and plant foods, but the animal sources are better absorbed and used by your body. Fish, poultry, lean meats, eggs, nuts, seeds and dried beans and peas are good staple protein foods. So is soy (as in tofu), but breast cancer survivors should probably limit soy, as it raises estrogen levels, which can be a risk for a cancer recurrence. Protein's primary function is to build new body structures (like muscles and organs), heal damaged structures and replace worn-out cells. It can also serve as a source of energy, but you don't want to waste protein on a job that's really better suited to carbohydrates. By eating enough carbohydrates, we allow protein to be devoted to the building work it does best.

Vitamins and Minerals are really two separate categories, but I will combine them here because they serve similar roles in the body. I nickname them "the assistants" because they help with a variety of functions of your body. For example, vitamin A helps with eyesight; vitamin D, calcium and phosphorus (both minerals) help build bones; vitamin C aids in immunity; and iron helps red blood cells carry oxygen throughout the body. A wide variety of foods feature different minerals and vitamins, which is why it's a good idea to eat from all of the food groups and to choose different types of foods within each group. Aim to eat lots of different colors of foods; it's a simple strategy, but effective.

By the way, vitamins and minerals do not contain calories; therefore, they do not give us energy in the true sense of the word. The B vitamins help us use our energy sources, but supplements of them cannot make up for an inadequate diet.

Water is the nutrient found in greatest abundance in the body, and it's the one we can live without for the least amount of time. It does several major jobs in the body, but the most important thing to remember is that every bodily process happens in the presence of water and probably can't happen if water isn't present. You need to drink at least 8 cups of water a day, and that's a conservative estimate.

Where do calories come from?

We find calories in carbohydrates, fat and protein. Carbohydrates and protein each contribute 4 calories in one gram, and fat contributes 9 calories in one gram. Put another way, a teaspoon of sugar contains 14 calories and a teaspoon of butter or oil contains 33 calories. Alcohol contributes 7 calories in one gram, which your body promptly turns into fat and stores it in your abdomen, hence the term "beer gut." Fiber passes through the body undigested, so it doesn't contribute any calories. None of the other nutrients contain calories, either.

The amounts of carbohydrate, fat and protein you should eat each day, according to the experts

There is a LOT of debate over how much carbohydrate, fat and protein you should eat each day. The number of grams you eat will vary according to your calorie needs, so the experts give you the recommendations as percentages. In other words, of your total calorie consumption for a day, a certain percentage should come from each of the three macro-nutrients (the three nutrients that contain calories – carbohydrate, protein and fat). If you eat 2,000 calories a day and you are aiming to get 50% of your calories from carbohydrates, then you would eat 1,000 calories worth of carbohydrate, which is 250 grams (1,000 divided by 4 equals 250). Confused? The website freedieting.com has a nutrient calculator in its tools section to help you figure out your exact numbers based on the calories you eat per day. In general, the professionals recommend that you eat anywhere from 45 – 65% of your calories from carbohydrate, 20 – 30% of your calories from fat, and 15 – 35% of your calories from protein.

MY DIET IS BASED ON SIX MAIN PRINCIPLES

I've never been a fan of nutrition programs that include detailed menus and recipes. There are some great ones available and you may find them helpful, but I prefer to know the philosophy behind the diet and then have the flexibility to choose my own foods based on that knowledge. My eating philosophy is summarized in six key ideas.

1. **Vegetables are the foundation of my diet.** Every day, I eat combinations of broccoli, mushrooms, asparagus, spinach, lettuce, cabbage, tomatoes, onions, summer squash, Brussels sprouts, and similar lower-carbohydrate choices. In smaller amounts, I eat carrots, sweet potatoes and winter squash, as they are higher in carbohydrates, yet still very nutritious. Vegetables are a staple of most meals, and I have developed creative ways to replace starches, such as white potatoes, bread and pasta, with these more nutrient-dense choices. They are high in fiber, vitamins and minerals, and they provide a sense of fullness without contributing a lot of calories. Shredded zucchini, lightly browned in a little olive oil, makes a great substitute for pasta. Steamed spinach is delicious with marinara sauce; I skip the pasta in favor of spinach, and I enjoy it just as much.

2. **I eat enough protein.** There's a legitimate debate over the amount of protein you should eat in a day. Proponents of diets with only 15% of your calories coming from protein (about two 3-ounce servings of meat, fish or poultry a day) claim that your body doesn't need more than this, that too much protein is dangerous to your health, and that many protein foods also contribute unhealthy fats. They also point to the ecological and moral ramifications of eating a diet high in animal products; it uses far more natural resources to raise beef than it does to raise grains, and the way in which commercial animals are raised seems cruel to many of us (myself included). These are all valid arguments, and I think they have merit. In fact, I spent years of my life prior to cancer as a vegetarian and enjoyed those years.

Yet, after my cancer diagnosis, I decided to increase my protein to about 35% of my daily calories. I made this choice for several reasons. First, I was diagnosed with iron-deficiency anemia a year prior to having cancer, and adding animal products was an important part of the remedy for me. I also knew that my body needed more protein to aid in my recovery from cancer treatment. Finally, as a figure contestant, eating enough protein is essential for building muscle. While I'm not a strong advocate for supplements, I use a whole protein supplement after my training sessions. I no longer eat tofu and other soy-based protein, as my cancer was estrogen-sensitive and eating soy can promote estrogen production

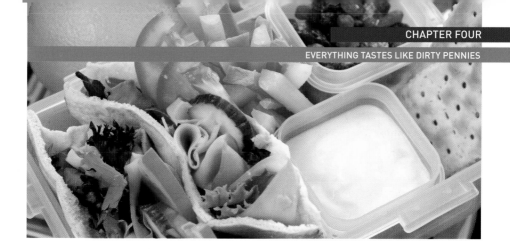

in my body. My primary dietary sources of protein include plain, nonfat Greek yogurt; fish, egg whites and poultry. I've found a farm near me where I can buy locally-raised poultry and eggs. I have also become a fan of hunted deer meat (as opposed to farm-raised) when I can get it. The challenge is that hunters are not allowed to sell their meat, so I have to find donated sources. I love hunted deer meat for two reasons. First, it is an ecologically sound and humane way to get meat and, second, it's leaner and higher in protein than commercially raised meat.

3. **I eat whole, unprocessed foods as much as possible.** Fresh food tastes better and allows me greater control over the amount and type of fats, sugar, sodium and other things I want to limit. It's more nutrient-dense and I'm less likely to binge on these kinds of foods than I am on processed foods.

4. **I devote time each day to preparing my meals and packing food to take with me.** At first, it took a lot of time and thought to pack foods to take to work and on trips (day trips or overnight). As I developed a routine for it, it became a faster and simpler process. I purchase very few meals, preferring to pack my lunch (and sometimes dinner, too) for work; visits to the zoo, museum, or beach with my kids; and long car rides. Each night, I take time to consider my schedule the following day and then pack the appropriate foods I want to take with me. I store them in the refrigerator in travel containers that I bring home and reuse. I try to limit restaurant dining to about once a month, and I reserve this for a meal that I will enjoy and is special, such as dinner out with my husband. When staying in a hotel, I will go to a grocery store for fresh fruit and vegetables that don't need refrigeration, peanut butter and wheat bread to eat for snacks.

5. **I eat low glycemic load foods and as little sugar and flour (even whole wheat) as possible.** I love sweets, cakes and breads! I would eat bread, cake, cookies and chocolate several times a day if they had no ill effect on my energy or body fat levels. The problem is that sugar and flour stimulate my appetite; the more I eat, the more I want. It's very hard for me to have one, tiny piece of cake and be satisfied, so I have developed an alternative strategy to satisfy my sweet tooth without setting myself up for undue temptation and overeating.

Before I share that strategy, I want to explain the value of low glycemic load foods and why it's helpful to me to follow this eating principle. Glycemic load refers to the amount and type of sugar found in a food and the effect this has on your blood sugar level after you eat this food. Foods with a high glycemic load are more likely to cause a quick rise and fall in your blood sugar, causing you to feel hungry again soon after you eat them. Low glycemic load foods provide a slower change in your blood sugar and allow you to feel full and satisfied for a longer period of time. Through experience, I've learned that I am sensitive to the glycemic load of foods. As a figure contestant, I want to keep my body fat low, so it's particularly important for me to not overeat, particularly carbohydrates.

How do I satisfy my daily desire for something sweet without triggering a sugar binge? After weighing the evidence, I decided to use the artificial sweeteners sucralose (the brand name is Splenda, but you can buy cheaper generic versions) and the plant-based Stevia. The use of artificial sweeteners is one of the more controversial topics in nutrition. You may decide to not use them, particularly as a cancer survivor, and I understand your decision. Having small amounts of sugar may have no adverse effects on you, which could make sugar a good option for you.

I have created two simple dessert recipes using either sucralose or Stevia. I only add cinnamon and vanilla to non-fat, plain Greek yogurt and find that I don't miss a sweetening effect. The recipes are not gourmet, but they are simple, fat-free, sugar-free, and relatively low in carbohydrates and have a low glycemic load. In other words, I can eat them on a regular basis. Unlike sugar, these sweeteners don't cause a spike in my blood sugar and make me want to eat more sugar or starch.

How to choose low glycemic load foods

You may be familiar with the term glycemic index and wonder why I am referring to glycemic load instead. They are not the same. Glycemic index simply tells you how quickly a food will raise your blood sugar level based on the type of sugar it contains. Glycemic load gives you a fuller picture by also factoring in the amount of sugar found in a food, which is why I prefer to look at the glycemic load of a food.

Low glycemic load foods include whole grain products, such as pumpernickel and barley breads, whole wheat bread (especially if it is coarsely milled); tomato juice; All Bran breakfast cereal; most dairy products (except yogurt if sugar has been added); grapefruit, apples and watermelon; dried beans, nuts and seeds; meat, fish and poultry; and non-starchy vegetables, such as broccoli, lettuce, and carrots.

High glycemic load foods include processed foods in general, white potatoes, most breakfast cereals, white bread, anything made with a lot of sugar, bagels, white or brown rice, bananas, and most fruit juices.

There are many other foods that could be added to either of these lists, so it's worth it to find a bigger list of foods (free on the internet) if you are interested. There are a few surprises, too. Green bananas have a lower glycemic load than do ripe bananas. Brown rice has a higher glycemic load than white rice. Pretzels have a higher glycemic load than potato chips. Finally, fruit roll-up candy has a higher glycemic load than M & Ms, a Snicker's bar, popcorn or corn chips! In other words, it's best not to make assumptions about whether a food is higher or lower in glycemic load, but to check it out specifically.

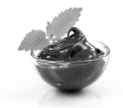

Two tasty sugar-free,
fat-free dessert recipes with nutrition facts.

Dark Chocolate Pudding

+ 1/2 cup dark cocoa powder
+ 2 tbsp. cornstarch
+ 1/4 cup sucralose (i.e., Splenda) or Stevia
+ 1/2 tsp. salt
+ 2 cups skim milk (I used lactose-free milk)
+ 2 tsp. vanilla extract

Blend the dry ingredients in a non-stick pot with a cooking spoon. Add one cup of the cold milk and stir until blended. THEN turn the stove on to medium heat and stir in remaining milk. Stir constantly until mixture boils. Let boil for one minute or until pudding thickens. Remove the pot from the heat and stir in the vanilla. Divide into four 1/2-cup servings and refrigerate until chilled.

Each 1/2 cup serving contains 70 calories, 5 grams of protein, 13 grams carbohydrate and less than one gram of fat.

Angel Food Cake

+ 12 egg whites (you can use a one-pint carton of egg whites and the cake will taste fine, but it won't be light and fluffy)
+ 1 cup flour
+ 2 cups sucralose (i.e., Splenda) or Stevia
+ 2 tsp. cream of tartar
+ 2tsp. vanilla extract
+ 1 tsp. almond extract
+ 1/2 tsp. salt

Set oven to 325 degrees. Put egg whites and cream of tartar in a mixing bowl and mix on low speed for 30 seconds. Then beat the mixture on high speed, slowly adding one cup of the sucralose/Stevia. Add vanilla and almond extracts and the salt. Continue to beat on high speed for at least 3 minutes, or until the mixture becomes stiff and forms peaks. Be patient and remember that, if you used a carton of egg whites, the mixture may not stiffen. After 3 minutes at high speed, turn off the mixer and slowly stir in the flour and remaining sucralose/Stevia by hand. Lightly coat a tube or bundt pan with cooking spray and pour in the batter. Bake for approximately 30 minutes. The cake is ready when the top is slightly brown and firm. After you remove it from the oven, immediately flip the pan over to remove the cake and allow it to cool (or not; sometimes I eat it hot!)

When cut into 14 pieces, each piece has 61 calories, 5 grams of protein, 10 grams of carbohydrate and less than one gram of fat.

I minimize foods that detract from my fitness goals or cause discomfort. Since cancer, I have developed irritable bowel syndrome (IBS), which is characterized by episodes of moderate to severe intestinal cramping and bloating and is compounded by constipation. For this reason, I have to limit or avoid foods that could be included in a healthful diet, such as dried beans. Dairy fats, such as those in ice cream and cheese, also trigger IBS in me, but the high saturated fat content of these foods alone is a reason for me to not eat them. My favorite

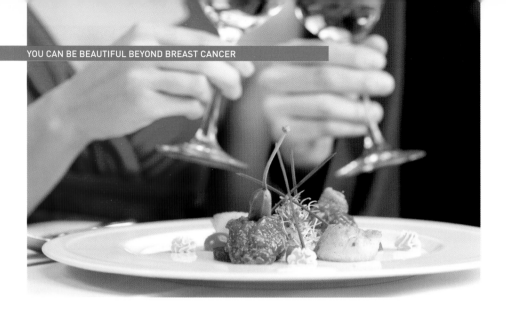

sources of fats are avocados, natural peanut butter, and olive or peanut oil used in cooking. While whole wheat grains, brown rice and oatmeal are very nutritious, I eat a little less of them now as I train for figure competitions. Too many starches lead to increases in body fat.

My grocery list. Here is a list of a typical week of grocery shopping for me. This list only represents what I eat, and not my husband and sons, who don't follow as strict a diet as I do. It does not represent everything I eat, but includes the foods I eat about 90% of the time.

I pack my lunch for work and eat in a restaurant about once a month.

Note: I try to follow the 90% rule, which means that I eat the above diet 90% of the time. About 10% of the time, I will have small portions of sweets and snacks. I don't buy these for myself, though, and try to limit them to social occasions or when I really have a craving for one.

My typical daily diet. Here is what I eat in an average day. My diet consists of six small meals a day, each one containing protein and fiber, in addition to carbohydrates, most of which have a lower glycemic load. It's important to note that everyone's caloric needs are unique, and I had to experiment before finding the right amount of food for me to maintain my weight and allow for muscle growth.

My Grocery List

- 3 quarts of Plain non-fat Greek yogurt
- half gallon of lactose-free skim milk
- One dozen eggs (I usually just eat the whites)
- 4 five-ounce cans of white tuna in water
- One pound sliced turkey breast
- 3 pounds of a white fish (like tilapia)
- 3 pounds of chicken breasts
- Whole protein powder (whey or egg-based)
- 2 heads green or red leaf lettuce
- 1 head cabbage
- 3 onions
- 2 bunches broccoli
- 4 tomatoes
- 1 pound green beans
- 4 sweet potatoes
- 1 bag fresh spinach
- 1 head cauliflower
- 4 bell peppers
- 2 grapefruit

- 1 pint each blackberries and blueberries
- 2 cantaloupe
- 1 pound mushrooms
- 4 summer or zucchini squash
- 1 bunch of celery
- fresh herbs (cilantro, dill, oregano)
- 1 avocado
- old fashioned oatmeal
- natural peanut butter
- 2 cans chicken broth
- 1 can garbanzo beans
- 5 low-carb multi-grain wraps
- Olive and peanut oil
- Balsamic vinegar
- Peanuts
- Black and green tea
- decaffeinated coffee
- 1 pint egg whites (for Angel Food Cake)
- Stevia or sucralose
- Cheerios, Corn Chex or Rice Chex (for post-training carbohydrates)

Meal 1:

+ 1 cup Greek non-fat yogurt (with added vanilla extract and nutmeg or cinnamon)
+ 1 cup berries
+ 1 cup cooked oatmeal in water with 1 tbsp. skim milk
+ 2 cups of black tea with 2 tbsp. skim milk, water

I often do my weight training after meal 1.

Meal 2:

+ 1.5 scoops of protein powder with 1 cup water and 5 ice cubes in a blender
+ 1 cup of a higher glycemic load cereal (like Corn Chex or Cheerios)

This is my post-training recovery meal to help my body absorb and use protein.

Meal 3:

+ 4 cups of vegetable stir-fry with egg whites
+ 1 low-carb wrap

Meal 4:

+ 3 cups green salad with vegetables and 5 ounces of white tuna, balsamic vinegar

Meal 5:

+ 5 – 8 ounces of fish or chicken, 2 cups cooked vegetable (such as broccoli), 1 cup cantaloupe

Meal 6:

+ 4 slices of turkey in a low-carb wrap with vegetables;
+ 1-2 servings of a sugar-free dessert

"Free" snacks:

Dill pickles or cut up vegetables (peppers, celery). I will also have 1 to 3 bites of sweets or snacks during the day, and I'm pretty good about limiting them to just a taste. A few times a year, someone will give us a bottle of wine, and I may have 2 ounces at night until it's gone, but I limit alcohol in my diet.

THE TWO THINGS YOU WON'T WANT TO DO AND WHY YOU SHOULD DO THEM ANYWAY

Of the six key ideas above, the hardest for most people to follow is making your own food and resisting the temptation to rely on frozen entrees, fast food, deli markets and other sources of already prepared food on a regular basis. Yet, of the six principles above, this is probably the most critical to me in maintaining a lean, strong, healthy body.

By preparing my food myself, I am able to follow the other five principles much more consistently and with less stress. I've learned that, to make this work for me, I have to do my planning at night for the next day. I will think through the following day's schedule at night and determine how much food I'll need to take with me, often cooking a stir fry and making a salad at 8 p.m. to pack for the next day. Nighttime cooking for the next day's meals has become a habit for me, and I no longer find it burdensome, nor do I forget to do it. Another strategy is to double the amount of what I am preparing one day and packing half of it away for the next day. This step is well worth the effort you will put into it. I am convinced that I would not have succeeded in cultivating a competition-ready body if I didn't make my own food.

A second activity you will be tempted to skip is tracking and analyzing your diet for a period of time. To do it effectively, you need to record everything you eat and drink throughout the day, every day for at least a week to see an accurate picture of your diet. The more accurately you record your food intake, the more useful the resulting analysis will be to you. This is an essential first step to knowing how to change your diet in order to get the results you want. How will you be able to create a strategy for change if you don't know your starting point? Once you do set goals for the type and amount of foods you want to eat, how will you know if you are meeting them unless you keep a record? You also won't know how nutritious your diet is unless you analyze it. There are several good computerized programs for tracking and analyzing your diet, and you can find several for free on the internet. A side benefit of recording your diet is that you will eat a more healthful one simply because you are writing it down. I'm more intentional about what I eat during the weeks I record my diet. (I don't record every week of my life; that would drive me crazy! I cycle in and out of recording my foods, making an attempt to follow my guidelines whether I am recording my diet or not.)

When you begin to record your diet, I encourage you to follow your normal eating habits during the first week to see how nutritious it is at the start. Then, following the goal-setting guidelines I provide in Chapter 5, I suggest you make one or two changes each week to bring your diet in line with what you would like it to be. If you would like more direction in planning your diet, I encourage you to invest in a few sessions with a registered dietitian or follow a professionally developed nutrition plan.

My favorite commercial nutrition program and why I recommend it

Are you interested in following a more specific nutrition program that will help you map out what you should eat and how much, as well as provide you with recipes and meal plans? If so, I recommend the Precision Nutrition (PN) program by Dr. John Berardi. Of all the commercial programs available for purchase, PN is the best I've reviewed for several reasons. First, it's based on sound nutrition principles and solid research. Second, it's very user-friendly, with great explanations of the plan, realistic daily strategies, suggestions to incorporate it into your life when you are pressed for time, and menu/meal plans. Third, PN doesn't make promises it can't keep; if you follow it, you really will reap the benefits it offers. Finally, Dr. Berardi's website offers a number of great features and resources to support you as you make this eating plan a permanent way of life.

FOLLOWING THIS PLAN AND ENJOYING A SOCIAL LIFE

My husband has made a serious hobby out of cooking gourmet Mexican food. As much as our schedules allow, we have dinner guests and Stuart will prepare a memorable meal for them. The recipes he prepares are made from fresh, whole ingredients, but it's a lot of food and can be higher in fat and carbohydrate than what I intend to eat, particularly if I am in a phase of training when I want to lower my body fat. I have heard of people who can sit in front of a gourmet spread and eat a few bites, but I am not one of them. How do I handle the temptation? I've developed a few strategies to help me be a gracious hostess, show my husband that I appreciate his fine cooking and enjoy the meal without eating more than I want to eat. First, I get up a lot from the table. I fill water glasses, heat up additional tortillas, clear dishes and put on the coffee. Physically getting

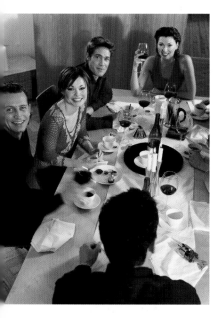

away from the food and being busy with a task keeps me from overeating. Second, I eat a lot of salsa, as it's made from tomatoes, tomatillas and other low-carbohydrate ingredients. I'll skip the cheese-covered beans and have a small amount of guacamole. Third, I make substitutions. One of my favorites is using strips of bell pepper instead of chips to dip into those low calorie salsas. At the end of the meal, I tell Stuart how wonderful the grilled fish with salsa was so that he is more likely to cook it again for me, ensuring that there will always be foods on the table that I want to eat.

Chances are, some of you are pretty social and like going out for drinks or meals with your friends every week. Maybe you are invited to people's homes for dinner or enjoy family gatherings over a meal. Good for you! Food is meant to give us pleasure and bring us together with the people we love. It facilitates celebrations, friendship, romance and other wonderful life experiences. The last thing I want to suggest is that you miss out on these experiences because you don't want to eat the food that's served. It's a struggle for me, though, to find the balance between enjoying food-based social activities and eating the way I want to eat. I'm certain that I don't get it right sometimes, but there are a few guidelines I follow to help me be gracious and fun to be around.

If someone has prepared a meal for me, I eat as much of it as I can. When people invite me to dinner, I've become a little bolder about telling them that, due to my health, there are a few foods I can't eat. I like to know this ahead of time when I'm cooking a meal for someone, so I figure other hosts might feel the same way. I try to keep this list short and uncomplicated for the host. If I'm going out to a restaurant, I'll often suggest Thai, Chinese, Japanese or Middle Eastern food. A good meal choice in Asian restaurants is steamed chicken and vegetables minus the sauce it is normally cooked in. I'll just add a little soy sauce at the table. If I'm in the mood to splurge on one menu item, such as dessert or garlic bread, I will conserve on my other choices and have salad without dressing and grilled fish without sauce. I avoid chain restaurants as much as possible; the food usually

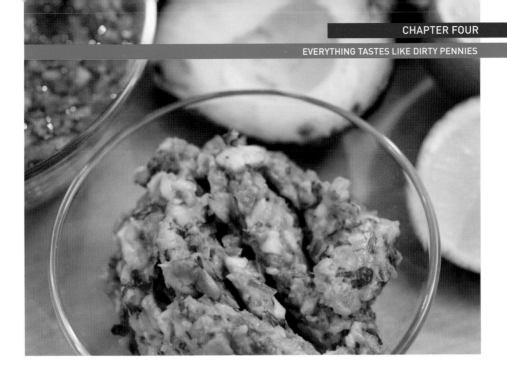

isn't as fresh, tasty or healthful as authentic ethnic foods. When I want to have lunch with a colleague, I'll frequently eat something ahead of time so I'm not too hungry at the restaurant and then order just a salad or soup. When planning time together with friends, I'll suggest that we meet at a park for a walk instead of meeting for a meal, or I'll invite them to my home for lunch or tea and coffee. Above all else, I don't talk about my diet or criticize the food that others are eating. I'd be such a bore and would ruin everyone else's fun! I eat the way I do because I *want* to, not because I feel that I must or should. I want my friends and family to feel the same freedom and look forward to spending time with me.

WHAT TO EAT TO PROMOTE HEALING AFTER SURGERY

There are two things to keep in mind when choosing what to eat after surgery. The first is that anesthesia and pain medication (like Percocet and Vicadin) can cause constipation, and it's a good idea to begin eating high fiber foods (and consider taking a laxative if your surgeon agrees) starting with your first post-surgery meal. Hospital food is not high in fiber; I brought a fiber supplement with me to the hospital and drank it every day, along with a lot of water. It's hard to get to the toilet with an IV in your arm, but I drank the water anyway. I also weaned myself off of the prescription pain killers and onto ibuprofen as soon as I could tolerate it, in part to minimize constipation.

The second thing to focus on after surgery is eating extra protein. Every cell in your body is made of a protein foundation, and protein is needed to generate the thousands of new cells needed to heal the surgical site, fight infection and maintain the rest of your body systems while you recuperate. My rule of thumb after surgery was to eat at least three servings of fish or chicken each day, along with skim milk and whole grains at each meal. Dark green and orange vegetables and citrus fruits will supply vitamins A and C and many other nutrients, which are also needed for healing.

EATING WELL THROUGH CHEMOTHERAPY

Chemotherapy symptoms are unique, according to just about all of the cancer survivors I've known. They are similar to having the flu, a migraine or a stomach ache, but not exactly the same. There are phases of treatment when I didn't want to eat anything, and other phases when I wanted to constantly eat foods like peanut butter and bread to settle my stomach. Foods taste different, too, with former favorites losing their appeal and new foods becoming more palatable. My sense of taste and smell were both affected. Foods containing sugar tasted metallic (like dirty pennies, someone aptly noted) and strong smells were nauseating.

Some women lose weight through chemotherapy and others gain weight. My goal was to maintain my weight, keeping as much lean body mass as possible. If you are overweight, chemotherapy is not the time to try to lose that excess fat unless your oncologist specifically recommends that you do so. I experimented with my diet after each cycle and, by cycle 3, had figured out the best eating plan to help me feel better and move through the symptoms faster while maintaining my weight. I still felt lousy much of the time but not as bad as I could have felt.

During the first few days after a chemotherapy treatment, I would wake up naturally at 2 a.m. or so and go into the kitchen for a small bowl of Shredded Wheat'n Bran cereal with skim milk and two 12-ounce glasses of water. Shredded Wheat'n Bran is one of the few cereals with no sugar added, so I could tolerate the taste of it better than other cereals. I didn't always want the water, but putting lots of ice in it and drinking it slowly helped get it down. This middle-of-the-night

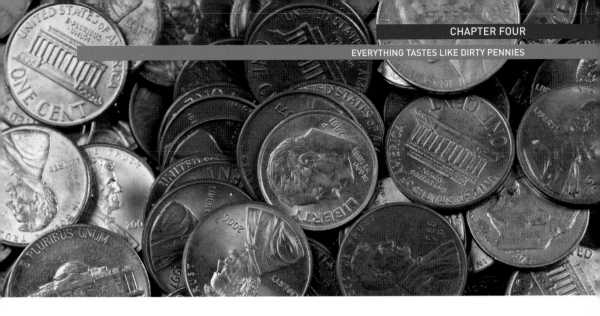

snack helped me feel less queasy in the morning. Drinking as much water as I could the first few days helped rid my body of the chemotherapy drugs faster, enabling me to feel better, even though it was hard to make myself do it. Some women are able to drink ginger ale more easily than water, but that was not the case for me. Ice water was the easiest beverage to drink without getting sick, so I sipped it all day.

As much as possible, I limited sodium in my diet, as it only made me feel worse. I ate small, frequent meals with minimal spices, sugar or fat in them. Too much fat or oil in a food would make me feel worse after eating it. There were days I was tempted to overeat in an effort to settle the queasy feeling in my stomach, but I soon learned that this caused intestinal pain. Eating very small amounts of food every hour or two was my best strategy. Oatmeal, Shredded Wheat'n Bran, bananas, turkey sandwiches, chicken soup, and baked chicken with roasted vegetables were the kinds of foods that I ate without feeling worse.

I also found it helpful to vary the foods I ate from one chemotherapy cycle to the next so that I didn't associate a particular food with my treatment. For example, someone gave us a pot of chicken soup during my first cycle and I found I could eat it fairly easily. Word got around, and soon lots of well-meaning friends were sending us pots of chicken soup after each chemotherapy treatment! By the third cycle, the sight of a pot of chicken soup made me feel nauseous even before I had my chemotherapy infusion because the soup was a reminder of the treatment to come. It was during that cycle that I added variety to my diet to prevent such associations.

By the 11th day of each chemotherapy cycle, I was feeling well again and could follow my six basic diet principles and engage in intensive fitness training. I had ten days to enjoy this before my next cycle of treatment.

IF MOMMA AIN'T HAPPY, AIN'T NOBODY HAPPY

It takes a special person to be successful at figure training. You have to be very determined and probably a little bit crazy, too, to follow such a demanding training and diet program. So far, I have described eating principles that can work for most people, especially cancer survivors. That can't be said of the typical figure training diet, unfortunately.

To be a successful, competitive figure contestant, you have to simultaneously build big muscles and strip your body of as much fat as possible. These two goals work against each other naturally, and figure contestants are on a constant quest for the perfect diet and training program that will help them do both. Many resort to dangerous tactics, and I have a tremendous amount of respect for the handful of contest winners who achieve their physiques through completely natural, sane strategies. Compared to men, I think it's a little easier for women to develop a stage-worthy body without resorting to crazy measures to get lean; women have the option of competing in the figure division, which prizes the slightly smaller, and definitely natural, feminine form. For men, though, bigger is always better, period.

The typical healthy weight American woman will have between 20% and 30% of her total body weight come from fat (the rest is water, muscles, bones, organs and other lean tissues). A competitive female figure contestant may have 10% or less of her weight come from body fat by competition day. She doesn't live this lean all year; she couldn't and still gain muscle, let alone feel and look good. Eight months before my competition (about six weeks after my hysterectomy), my proportion of body fat was 19% of my total weight. It was 16% by competition day, and, at 137 pounds, I weighed two pounds less than I did when I graduated from high school! By figure training standards, I was not quite lean enough to win a prize. But by my personal standards, I thought I looked great (if I can say that without sounding boastful) and knew that I could not have safely reached a lower level, at least not for this contest. I had decided ahead of time that I would be as competitive as possible without sacrificing my health or relationships with my husband and sons.

THE KETOGENIC DIET TRAP

I am not a fan of the Atkins Diet or anything that resembles it, yet this is the sort of diet that many figure contestants follow in the months prior to a show, and a few follow it as long as their bodies can take it. The Atkins Diet is probably the most famous of a category of diet plans that intentionally seek to reduce carbohydrates to a low enough level that, when your body is attempting to burn calories and must rely too much on fat, substances called ketones are produced. Ketones are byproducts of fat metabolism when there's not enough carbohydrate present to burn them completely to supply your body with energy. Your body considers them a toxin and excretes them in your urine. When you eat enough carbohydrates, you don't produce very many ketones. In a low-carbohydrate, high-protein diet, your ketone production increases significantly and your kidneys need to make more urine to get rid of the excess ketones. This is dehydrating and puts extra strain on your kidneys, leading to kidney pain and damage over time. A ketogenic diet is one that intentionally leads to excessive ketone production.

Why would anyone follow a diet like this? It has many proponents, including some with good credentials in health and medicine. People like this diet primarily because you will lose a lot of weight initially. If you've been struggling for years to lose weight unsuccessfully and try this approach, you will likely lose several pounds and a dress size or two within a few weeks. Figure contestants like this diet because it's really hard to lose weight when you are already lean, especially without losing muscle mass. They believe this diet plan is better than any other to give them that result, although I haven't found any credible evidence that this is true.

I eat a diet that is higher in protein and moderate in carbohydrates, but I stop short of putting myself into ketosis. During my "off season," or when I am not within four

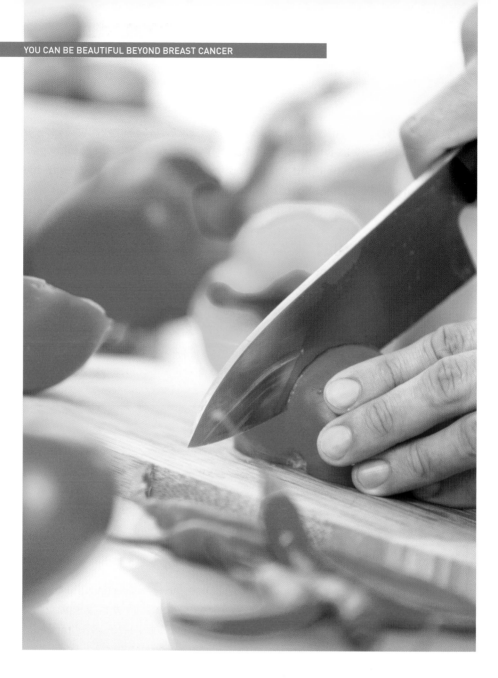

months of a competition, about 45% of my calories come from carbohydrates, 35% are from protein and the remaining 20% are from fat. Four months prior to the figure competition, I started reducing my calories overall to begin a slow weight loss process and ate an equal amount of protein and carbohydrate during that time period, with 40% of my calories coming from each. One month prior to the competition, I began working with a nutrition coach who encouraged me to reduce my carbohydrates slightly and increase the amount of protein I ate.

During these final four weeks, 35% of my calories came from carbohydrates, 44% from protein and 22% from fat. As an ongoing practice, I would not eat so few carbohydrates and so much protein. It's not healthy and it's not necessary for muscle growth or fat loss. In fact, I'm not sure if I will eat this way again as I prepare for future competitions, but I wanted to try it for the first one to see how my body responded. I found that the fewest number of carbohydrates I could eat in a day was about 130 grams without experiencing ketosis, and I learned through experience that ketosis is not something I can live with.

It started when I attempted to eat just 125 grams of carbohydrates for two days in a row, followed by two days of 150 grams and then back down to 125 grams for a day. After a week, I was miserable! I was swearing at the dog, grumping at my children and had no interest in sex with my husband. I also found that I had no enthusiasm for any of my usual interests. I concluded that the price I was paying to become a little bit leaner was not worth the unhappiness it caused me or my family, so I ate a few more carbohydrates to stay above my ketogenic level. I was doing this for personal fulfillment and enjoyment, after all! I knew that if this was going to be more than a one-time experience for me, I had to feel good about the preparation process.

IT'S CALLED EATING, NOT CHEATING

Remember at the beginning of the book, when I promised to share my failures and weaknesses, as well as my victories and strengths, with you? Well, it's time for me to share a weakness. While I don't qualify for an official diagnosis of anorexia nervosa, I have come to admit that I dance around the edges of disordered eating. What's deceptive is that my lifestyle seems so ideal and my self-disciple is the envy of others. I am highly motivated to train and eat well, although I fear fat gains and sometimes I don't eat enough. Author Michael Pollan refers to a new term called "orthorexia," which he defines as an "unhealthy obsession with healthy eating."[1] I also see this phenomenon in my students who take health classes, particularly those in nutrition. Like me, they want to think about, talk about and analyze food all day long – everything short of actually *eating* very much of it that falls outside the bounds of what they consider a perfect diet. I'm well aware that the diet component of figure training can feed into this unhealthy obsession of mine, and I need to take steps to recognize it and protect myself from it.

Solving my problem is not simple, though. Irritable bowel syndrome is a real threat to me, and there are days when I legitimately need to limit the type and amount of food I eat to avoid triggering an episode. This is a smart and healthy thing to do. What's *not* smart and healthy is when I avoid foods because of an overriding fear of gaining fat and losing muscle, even when I am already lean. I wish I could tell you that I've overcome this problem and how I did it, but I can't. I've taken a few steps in the right direction, though. A handful of people close to me have permission to ask me questions about my diet, weight and health, and hold me accountable for my eating habits. I've also chosen a trainer and a competition coach who are both promoters of healthy methods for losing body fat in preparation for a competition.

Finally, I am aware of my thoughts about food and even the language I use to describe what I eat and how I feel about it. Our culture engages in a lot of moralizing about food, which fosters unhealthy attitudes. Chocolate cake is not sinful or decadent, yet we frequently hear those adjectives to describe it. Eating dessert is not "cheating"; it is enjoying something that is meant to be pleasurable.

REFERENCES

1   Pollan, M. (2008). *In Defense of Food*. New York City, NY: The Penguin Press.

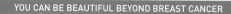

Melon raw
Milk 0% fat
Milk 0.5% fat
Milk 3.2% fat
Milk goat
Milk sheep
Mincemea
Mullberri
Muesli
Nectari
Oatme
Oil ve
Olive

3
255

2
940

10

615
120

740
66

2453

995
90
587
114

9

740
66
876
245
485
114

2392

740

16

740
72
759
202
40
476
112

23

CHAPTER FIVE

Failing to plan is planning to fail

CHAPTER 5

Failing to plan is planning to fail

I'm not an exercise physiologist or personal trainer, which is why I asked Domenick (who is both) to design the full training program that I used and the introductory portion of it that you will find in the appendix of this book. My expertise is in health behavior change. During the past 25 years as a health educator and, more recently, a certified wellness coach, I have helped hundreds of people lose weight, quit smoking, start exercise programs, end procrastination and make other changes important to them. Understanding why and how people make and maintain lifestyle changes is something that fascinates me, and I want to share my knowledge and experience concerning this critical component of a successful training and diet program with you.

Change is hard. Don't let anyone tell you otherwise. Fitness and nutrition programs that assure you of continuing to eat all your favorite foods and never feeling hungry, with just 15 minutes of exercise a day, are not the kind of programs that will give you the level of results I achieved. If your favorite foods are laden with sugar, white flour and fat and you want a leaner, more muscular body, you will need to find some new favorite foods. If you are overweight and want to lose some excess body fat, you will probably have moments of feeling a little hungry, and should choose to go outside for a walk instead of eating more food.

WHAT DO YOU REALLY WANT?

Because change is hard, it's important that you start by assessing yourself and answering the fundamental question "what do I really want to do with my time and energy?" Notice that this is different than the questions "what *should* I want?" or "what do *other people* think I should want?" The difference is that the second two questions are based on the premise of avoiding guilt and blame, as opposed to the first question, which guides you toward joy and fulfillment. I cannot think of a single client or student of mine who has made a lasting and

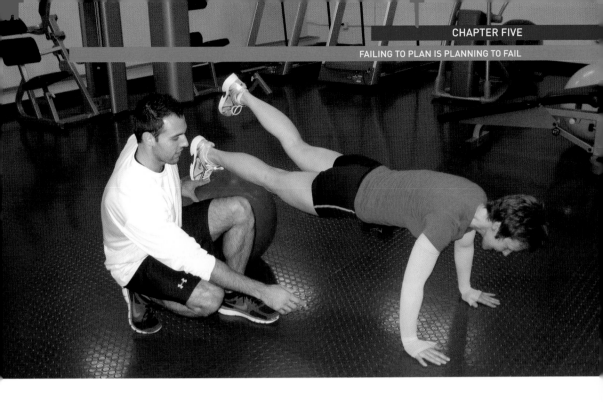

satisfying life change because she felt guilty about it or that she "ought" to do it. People can feel a lot of guilt concerning their diet and exercise habits, yet when this is the starting point for making a change, someone is less likely to have the motivation to succeed. As a wellness coach, I begin by asking my clients "what is your heart's desire?", "what would make you really happy?" and "what matters most to you?" It is for these things, and only these things, that you will pay the high price of creating something new in your life. Competitive figure training is something I want to do badly enough that I am willing to follow a challenging training program and carefully monitored diet almost every day of the year in order to be ready for competition. Plenty of times, I have said "no thanks" to a slice of cake that has tempted me, knowing that my ability to train effectively and stay lean matters more to me than the satisfaction of that dessert. I couldn't say no to the dessert otherwise.

What do you feel that strongly about? Please let me be straightforward and remind you that if you've had cancer, you don't have the luxury of putting off your dreams and desires forever, or allowing guilt and obligation push you toward doing things you don't really desire to do. What are you excited about? What is worth paying a high price to achieve? That's the best indication of where to set your goals now, and you can start working toward them in the process of cancer treatment.

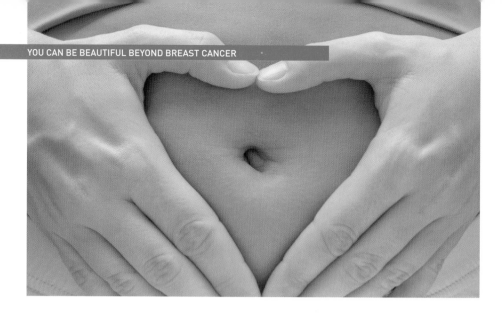

HOW TO GET WHAT YOU REALLY WANT

I'll assume that, since you've read this far, your desire is to achieve your fitness potential through a training program, a better diet, and perhaps other changes, too. Now you need to have a clear plan. I've found that the most successful plans are specific and concrete; in other words, they are spelled out in detail and tell you exactly what you need to do each day in order to follow them. In my experience, I have seen that people who have well-thought-out plans succeed and those with vague plans fail. Getting what you really want depends a lot on the quality of the plan you devise to achieve it, so please don't skim over this part. In this section, I want to share with you a tried-and-true, five-step approach to creating a plan that has worked well for me and for my students and clients.

STEP ONE:
Set SMART goals

A SMART goal is *Specific, Measurable, Action-oriented, Realistic,* and *Time-oriented.*[1] The best goal is the one that motivates you to want to reach it. It's specific, which means it's crystal clear, so you know exactly when you are meeting your goal and when you aren't. You've stated it in a way that makes it measurable, which means you can count up the number of times you do it in a day or a week. It's action-oriented, which means the goal focuses on a habit that you can control (like eating more vegetables), as opposed to an outcome that you may not be able to control (like losing five pounds this month). A realistic goal is one that you potentially could achieve, and not an impossible fantasy. Finally, you have a clear idea of when you will reach this goal, making it time-oriented.

Let me give you an example that is typical of what I've seen in my students and clients. I'll start with the not-so-effective goal and then show you how to make it SMART.

Not So Effective Goal: I want to fit into my skinny jeans again

What could possibly be wrong with this goal? It's written on at least half of the testimonials for diet plans and even a few breakfast cereal boxes. I'm not a big fan of this goal for two reasons. First, there's a chance this may be more of a fantasy than a reasonable expectation. If your skinny jeans are just one size smaller than the pair you are currently wearing, it might be realistic for you to get into them again. If you haven't worn your skinny jeans in the eight years since your kids were born and you are now several sizes larger, then it might be in the realm of fantasy. A good rule of thumb for identifying a target body weight you'd like to reach is to choose a weight that you have been able to comfortably maintain for at least six months during your adult life. If you have had children since you were at that target weight, you may need to readjust your expectations slightly. (For what it's worth, I am now at my high school graduation weight, but my waistline is still a little larger than it was before I had children. I feel great about my body, but it's different now than it was before my pregnancies.)

My second concern is that this not-so-effective goal focuses on an outcome, which is weight loss and size reduction, rather than a habit over which you have control. The important concept here is that we *don't have direct control over outcomes, only our behavior.* You can directly control whether you eat a bowl of ice cream for dessert or whether you exercise today. You *cannot* directly control whether you lose two pounds this week. I believe in setting *behavioral* goals because those are the ones you can control, so you have a great opportunity to be successful at them. You can do all of the right things, such as eating less food and exercising, but not lose two pounds this week. Why? Because weight loss is unpredictable in the short term and you don't have direct control over it. Over months of steady calorie restriction and exercise, you will lose weight, but it may happen at a pace that's different from the one you anticipated. If you focus on changing a behavior, then you are setting the stage to be successful at the end of the week and feel good about staying with that behavior. If you focus on reaching an outcome, such as losing a certain number of pounds, then you are more likely to feel like a failure at the end of the week, *even if you maintained some great eating and exercise habits that will eventually lead to weight loss*.

SMART version of this goal: I want to eat five small meals each day, with additional snacks limited to low-calorie vegetables (such as celery and cucumber slices). Each meal will contain approximately 300 calories and will include some vegetables, lean protein and fiber.

This goal works for several reasons. It's specific and measurable, which means that you know exactly what you're going to do and can clearly state at the end of a day whether you did it or not. It provides the average woman with a realistic number of meals and calories per day and focuses on your actions, which you can control. And if you set a reasonable time period in which to consistently eat this way, you will probably find yourself losing the weight and inches you had hoped to lose. Finally, you are more likely to stick with this goal because you have an opportunity to be successful every day; if you follow your diet and exercise plan, you can enjoy the feeling of accomplishment this brings at the end of each day, regardless of how much weight you lose in a given week.

STEP TWO:
Make your progress visible

It's amazing to me how many fifty-year-olds love sticker charts. I first learned this when I led programs to help clients quit smoking. They would take home a calendar and put a sticker on every smoke-free day they achieved. Many would later tell me that they continued using sticker charts for up to a year, and some even put a small, daily victory sign in their planners well beyond the first year. They weren't all kindergarten teachers, either. Business managers, firefighters, restaurant-owners and computer technicians were also part of this group, and some said that the daily reward of being able to put a sticker on the chart was the

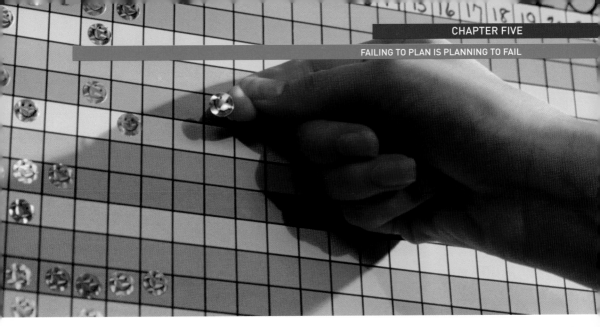

SINGLE most important strategy that helped them quit smoking. I think there's a lesson for all of us here, regardless of the habit we are trying to change. When your progress is clearly visible to you, it inspires you to keep working toward your goal.

How can you make your progress visible? You could take before-and-after photos, put stickers on a calendar, or track on a chart your gains in strength and endurance as you exercise. As I was preparing for my figure competition, I took photos of myself performing the competition poses every three months. It was thrilling to me to compare the photos over time and see the changes my body was making. Had I not taken the photos, I would not have been aware of how much I had achieved over time. I also keep a log each time I train with weights, noting the amount of weight I used and how many times I lifted it. I find great satisfaction in looking over my logs for the past year and seeing how much stronger I've become.

STEP THREE:
Say encouraging words to yourself all day long

Also called affirmation or positive self-talk, this is a necessary strategy that is often over-looked by otherwise committed, hard-working, goal-driven people. Why? Because they think they don't need it or, worse, that they shouldn't need it. Don't let some ill-conceived notion of positive self-talk being only for weaker women get in the way of you harnessing this powerful tool. We all say things to

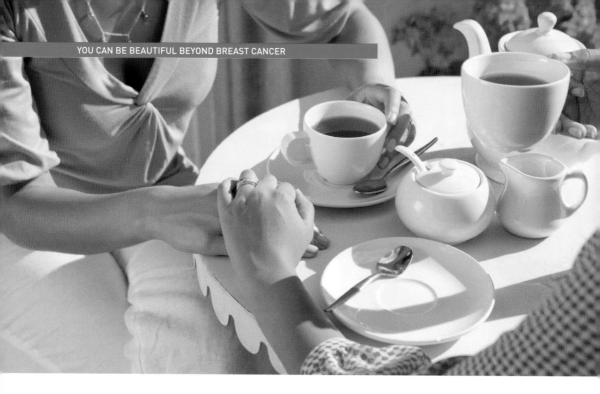

ourselves all day long, whether we are conscious of it or not. The trick here is to make this a conscious process and then choose the messages you want to say to yourself. I do it all the time and it helps me face my fear, calm down when I'm feeling anxious and just generally keep going when I feel like quitting. Imagine what you would say to a beloved friend if she were in your present situation and then tell that to yourself. When I'm feeling anxious, I remind myself that this anxious feeling will pass and I'll feel hopeful again tomorrow. If I am tired, I give myself permission to not have to make any tough decisions that day and offer myself small rewards (like sitting down for five minutes to drink a cup of tea) if I can just get through one task. And my all-purpose winning affirmation is to remember that God loves me and is with me in every situation. My self-talk messages may or may not work for you, so I encourage you to write a few of your own and then consciously say them to yourself several times a day.

STEP FOUR:
Find someone to hold you accountable

We are inherently social beings and thrive best when we are in relationships with others. Even the quietest among us needs to have at least one person with whom she can be close. You'll be much more likely to stay with your goal if you involve at least one other person in the process with you. This person might join you in making the change or simply be an encourager and someone to hold you accountable for doing what you said you were going to do. My one suggestion for this person is that she or he be a *positive* person in your life. You don't need anyone who will nag, shame or berate you. You DO need someone who will point out your strengths and successes, really listen to what you are saying and encourage you to make the best decisions for yourself.

STEP FIVE:
If one strategy isn't working, try a new one

Of the five steps I've shared in this section, I've saved what I think is the most important for last. A common, but false, belief is that in order to be successful, you have to stick with your original game plan and if you change the plan, then you have failed. Don't fall for this flawed thinking! It's right up there with the notion that winners don't need positive self-talk or support partners, and it will undermine your resolve and confidence in no time. **If your plan isn't working, then change the plan.** I encourage you to think of at least three strategies to help you stick with your new behavior, with full awareness that two of them probably won't work. That's o.k. Often, it just takes **one** good strategy to help you succeed. I've witnessed this in my students and clients many times over the years. Just one strategy that really worked was all it took for them to eat more vegetables, stretch every day, quit smoking or start a weight training program. Having someone else to help you brainstorm a new list of strategies is very helpful in this case and could be a great role for the accountability partner you identified in step four.

OVERCOMING A LACK OF MOTIVATION

Some of you are not sure if you are ready to make a change and begin a fitness and diet program. You might be lacking the motivation to try the five-step plan I shared in this chapter and feeling frustrated that you lack the desire to stick with a diet and exercise plan, even if it's a good one.

This is a good time for me to introduce you to Dr. James Prochaska, the creator of what is arguably the most popular and widely used lifestyle change theory around today.[2] It's called the Transtheoretical Model and includes a component that many refer to as "readiness to change." In his early research, Dr. Prochaska learned that, for any given bad habit, such as smoking or not exercising, a significant number of the people he studied knew they needed to change but were mentally not ready to change their habit right now. He called them "contemplators" because they were stuck in the place of wanting to change and *not* wanting to change at the same time. They spent months or years thinking about, or contemplating, the much-needed change without being able to do anything about it. Sound familiar? Most of us have been in this place at some point in our lives.

So Dr. Prochaska coined the term "readiness to change" as a way of assessing whether a person was ready to successfully take action and change their habit now, or if they were still contemplating it. He understood that these contemplators were frequently misunderstood as not caring or wanting to change, and he set out to help them. I spent five years doing research on the Transtheoretical Model, and I think there are some terrific insights in it to help contemplators build their motivation to making the change they want to make. Here's my summary of what works.

Insight One:
See yourself in a new way

Often when people change, there's a domino effect. One change leads to another, which leads to yet another. It just takes finding that first habit to successfully change that will lead to many more positive changes that you might not see at the start. Why does this happen? I think it has to do with how success changes your vision of who you are. Let me give you an example. Years ago, I had a student we'll call Diane who became the president of the student chapter of the professional society for students in our discipline. Diane saw this as an honor and as the culmination of all the steps she'd taken toward becoming a leader in our field. About a month into her term, Diane came to my office for what she said would be a serious conversation. "Dr. Spencer, I've been keeping a secret from you that

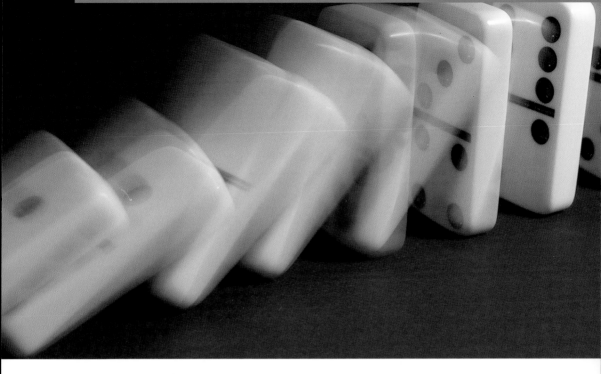

I just can't keep any more. I feel so lousy about it, and you may not want me to be the student chapter President after I tell you." What could she possibly have done? Turns out she was a weekend smoker. She worked as a hostess in a bar (you could still smoke in bars then) and found it impossible to quit with everyone smoking around her. But she was starting to experience *cognitive dissonance*, which is a fancy way of saying that she was holding two conflicting roles in her life – the health promotion leader vs. the weekend party smoker – and she had to resolve it one way or another. This cognitive dissonance is what propelled Diane into finally quit smoking for good; she liked the new vision of herself as a health promotion leader and professional so much that it was powerful enough to give her the push she needed to quit smoking.

So, what is your vision for yourself? Who are you becoming? What habits are getting in the way of you becoming that person? Where do you experience cognitive dissonance? Diane had to first become a student leader before she was ready to quit smoking. What changes might you have to successfully make that will pave the way for you to make a healthful diet and exercise part of your life? You might need to make some other changes first and *then* tackle your diet and exercise goals.

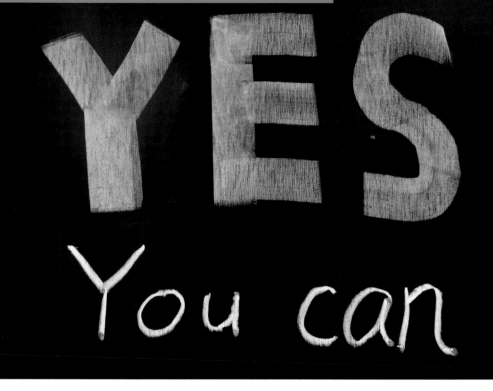

Insight Two:
Arouse your emotional energy

One mistake that health professionals like me can make is that we think people will change their habits simply because we tell them that their current way of doing things is unhealthy. We assume that all it takes is to give someone a list of the reasons why it's unhealthy to sit all day and eat too much processed food and that they will change. The truth is that they (like you) already know why these things are bad for them. Clearly, this is not enough to motivate a change in habits.

The problem with simply providing you with factual information about your health habit is that it only engages you on an intellectual level and ignores the emotional level altogether. While it's important to understand logically why the new habit is a good idea, you also need to *internalize* it by fully believing in your heart and soul that it is worth doing. To internalize it, you need to have feelings, and not just facts, about it. When we become emotionally engaged in making a change, we tap into a powerful source of energy. We think about it, care about it and talk about it whenever we can. We want to seek out other people who share our vision for it and collaborate with them. We get excited, and this excitement sustains us through the difficult work of making the change.

How do you arouse this emotional energy? You might read an inspirational story about someone who overcame adversity to succeed at something. Another strategy you might try is to create visual images that motivate you to want to change. An example of this is making a collage of images and phrases that inspire you and posting it where you'll see it often. You might also consider participating in a worthy cause, such as a walk to raise money for cancer research, to make your reasons for exercise more meaningful. Joining a club or class where you'll meet like-minded people with whom you can share this new passion is another great way to build your emotional investment in your new lifestyle.

Insight Three:
Weigh the benefits and the costs

Change always comes at a cost. If it didn't cost you something to change a bad habit, you would have already made the change. Don't make the mistake of telling yourself that there's nothing to like about the bad habit, because it's not true. You may find great comfort and reward at the end of a hard day by eating your favorite sweets and snacks in front of the television. Pretending that this isn't important does nothing to help you overcome it. Rather, it helps to make an honest and complete list of all the things you like about the current bad habit that you have. Allow yourself to feel how much you'll miss this bad habit and the good feelings it has given you. Then make a list of all the things you think you'll like about the new, good habits you plan to adopt. Again, put your heart into it as you imagine the many benefits that will come from your new lifestyle. You might want to do some reading or internet searching to learn more about these new habits so you can add to your list of potential benefits. Over time, the benefits of changing will become stronger and more important to you than the benefits you get from the current bad habit. It's at this point, and not until you reach this point, that you'll be ready to make the change. Instead of pushing yourself to make the habit change before you are ready, invest your time in building your list of reasons for changing to the new habit.

Dr. Prochaska and his colleagues have written an excellent, user-friendly book called *Changing for Good: A Revolutionary Six-Stage Program for Overcoming Bad Habits and Moving Your Life Positively Forward* (Avon Books, 1994) if you are interested in more in-depth reading on how to successfully change a habit. It provides a research-based approach to change in a format that's easy to read and apply to your life, with activities and worksheets to help you move toward your goal. It's my favorite among the self-help books for lifestyle change.

REFERENCES

1   I have most recently read the SMART goal acronym in the Circle Of Life wellness coaching leader's guide and participant handbook (www.col.com, 2012). While the idea probably didn't originate with them, I want to give them credit as my source for this great method of writing personal goals.

2   Prochaska, J. O., Norcross, J. C., DiClemente, C. C. (1994). *Changing for Good: A Revolutionary Six-Stage Program for Overcoming Bad Habits and Moving Your Life Positively Forward.* New York City, NY: Avon Books.

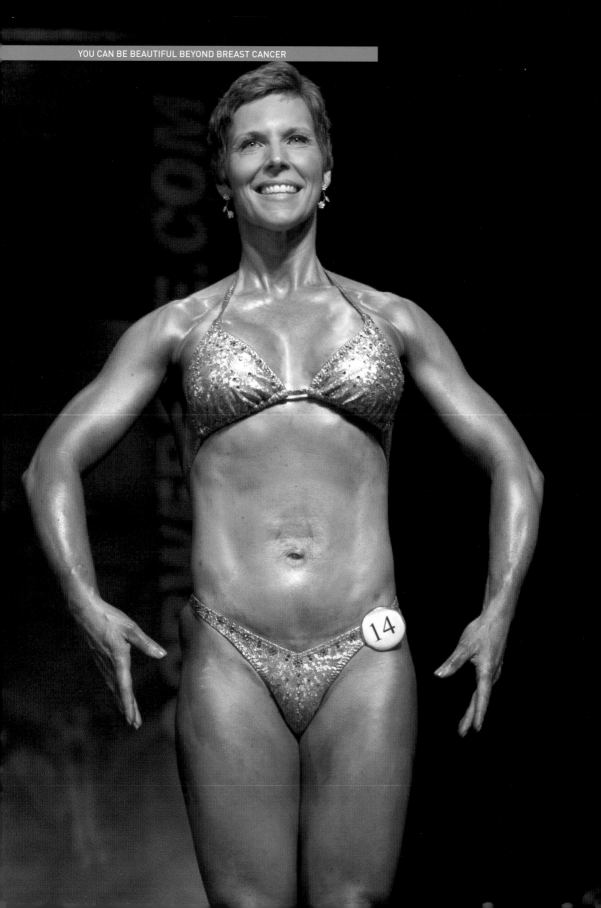

CHAPTER SIX

The beauty pageant with muscles

CHAPTER 6

The beauty pageant with muscles

There are many levels of physique contests like the one in which I participated. Most familiar would be bodybuilding, as it is the contest that men enter and was the first type of contest available to women. I participated in a figure competition. There is also a fitness model division (known as the bikini division in some organizations). I haven't made the distinction between these divisions yet, but it's a very important one for any female competitor. When women first entered the bodybuilding world in the late 1970s, they competed as did the men, performing the same poses and working toward the same goal of big muscles. As women's bodybuilding grew as a sport through the 1980s and 1990s, so did the size and shape of their muscles, displaying a level of development that is impressive but not desired by many women who wished to compete in this kind of contest. By the early 2000s, a new division called figure was created for female competitors who wanted to be judged by criteria that emphasized aesthetic appearance and symmetry of their physiques rather than muscle size. Figure competitors have observable muscles to be sure, but they are judged on the beauty, proportionality, and presentation of their physiques. Figure competitions have become enormously popular; in the competition I was in, there were five female bodybuilding contestants and over 30 figure contestants. This is typical of many competitions. Another newer division is fitness model, or bikini, and focuses even less on muscle development than does figure. What's valued in these competitions is stage presentation and looking great in a bikini and athletic wear. These competitions can launch careers in modeling fitness clothes and equipment. A final category is the fitness competition, in which contestants must perform a one-minute gymnastics/dance routine.

To the uninitiated, a figure competition looks like a bit of a spectacle. You see a group of women spray-tanned to the color of a pot roast, wearing high heels worthy of a stripper and tiny swathes of crystal-studded fabric, strike muscular poses while smiling like a Miss America contestant. The athleticism of the event and dedication of the athletes (yes, athletes) on stage is not self-evident to those

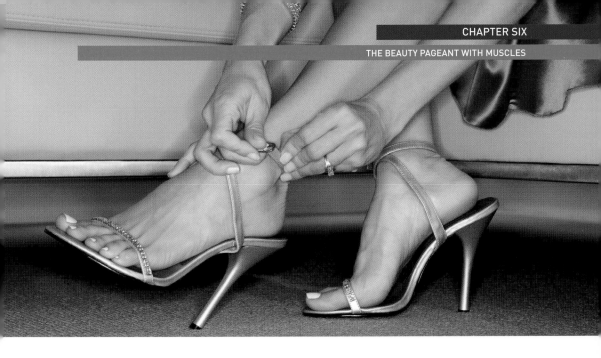

who are unfamiliar with bodybuilding. You might be tempted to think that the goal of the women on stage is to simply look sexy, and you would be wrong. Bodybuilding competitions are won based on the size and presentation of your muscles, not your breasts. When I competed, I was pleasantly surprised that we were admonished to avoid presenting ourselves in a provocative way; flirting with the judges would cause us to lose points, not earn them. We were reminded that we were athletes who had worked very hard to achieve our physiques and we were not to cheapen that by attempting to rely on sexual appeal on stage. Similarly, when I was shopping for a posing suit, I was pleased to learn that most contests prohibit contestants from wearing thong bikini bottoms. To be honest, I had expected that I would have to wear a thong bottom. While I have never been modest about my body, I wasn't quite sure I was ready to wear a thong bikini on a stage and was relieved to learn that it wasn't an expectation or even allowed in many contests.

A few people have expressed concern that, as the wife of a pastor, I should not be presenting myself publicly in such a revealing way. When I first considered entering a bodybuilding contest, I knew the potential for it to be negatively perceived by some members of the Christian community, both within and beyond our church. My husband and I discussed it, and he was fully supportive of my goal from the start. This prompted me to consider the conflicted ways in which we, as Americans, view our bodies and our sexuality. It extends beyond the religious community, although this is the group that simply may be more vocal about it.

In my opinion, we have lost the ability to appreciate the beauty and appeal of the human body without seeing it as an object of lust. Like paintings of nudes appreciated for their art, the presentation of oneself in a figure competition is an aesthetic expression, not a sexualized one.

PREPARING FOR A FIGURE CONTEST

So what's it like to be in a figure contest? What's involved in preparing for one? Allow me to enlighten you about this unique culture and why I am drawn to it. Let me begin by saying that preparing for a figure contest is plain old hard work, but the benefits far outweigh the cost for me.

Posing, or what those guys at the gym are doing in front of the mirrors

One unexpected benefit of contest preparation is that the combined practice of stage walking and posing has improved my posture and the way I carry my body. I stand taller, move more gracefully and hold myself with more poise since I've begun this practice. Posing is a habit that I practice on a near-daily basis all year round. You've probably seen those guys at the gym who love to flex their muscles in front of the mirror after every exercise they do. I used to think they were just vain and self-absorbed, but now I understand that they were practicing body-building poses. (Of course, some of them may still be vain and self-absorbed!) Figure contestants strike four poses on stage – front, right side, rear, and left side – separated by quarter turns of the body. It was through posing in front of a mirror that I discovered my tendency to round my shoulders forward. Now I'm in the habit of rolling my shoulders back, and I consistently look and feel taller and leaner. Another habit I practice on a regular basis is stage-walking. You might be surprised at the amount of time a figure contestant spends learning how to walk across a stage in four-inch heels. I practiced this twice a week for the four months prior to the show, and I would have liked to practice more had I been able to find a large-enough space to walk in every day. Watching You Tube instructional videos helped me to refine my gait. I learned to take longer strides, walk in a straight line, and to slow my pace, allowing me to glide more as I move.

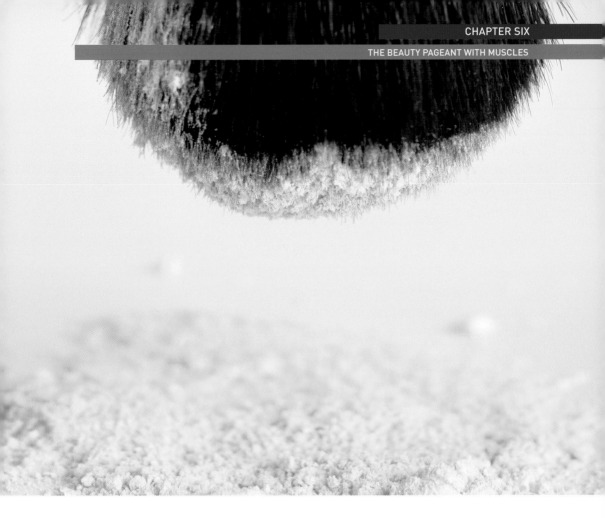

Posing suits: The thousand-dollar bikini you can't swim in

Another interesting, if not slightly stressful, experience was finding a posing suit. Some initial internet searching showed me that I could spend anywhere between $80 and $1,500 on a posing suit, I could rent or buy one, and if I bought one, I could get it used or new. Wow – there was a lot to figure out with this suit!

I learned that a posing suit is not the same as a bikini (even a bikini designed for stage contests), and that each contest-sponsoring organization has rules about how figure suits need to fit your body, particularly the cut of the suit bottom. Contestants are usually looking for high-impact suits that will sparkle under the stage lights. As a result, most suits have varying amounts of crystals glued on them, and it's the number and type of crystals that have the most influence on the cost of the suit. I ended up spending $250 on a custom-made suit by Tracy Edwards, a designer in North Carolina, and was immensely pleased with its look and cut. Tracy helped me get the most "bling" for my buck; she suggested a silver-dusted fabric, which gave the suit a lot of shimmer while using fewer crystals.

Fake tans, fake eyelashes and fake boobs… all parts of a "natural" competition

Figure contests pride themselves on being "all natural," which means that the competitors have achieved their physiques through natural, legal means and not by taking steroids. Some contests enforce this qualification with more rigor than others. The contest I was in was very thorough in its drug screening, which increased the chances that the competitors were presenting bodies they had developed through hard work and good genetics (thanks Mom and Dad), and not through questionable methods. The big joke, however, is that aside from our naturally developed muscles, the rest of our "look" is definitely fake.

For starters, we all sported something called a competition tan, which is an intensely dark spray-on tan that you would otherwise never wear in public. You have to start applying the spray tan a day or two ahead of time in order to get enough layers of the stuff on your skin. Most contestants will stay indoors during those two days, wearing long sleeves and pants (even in the summer) to keep the tanning solution from getting on other fabrics and surfaces. Being this dark shows off our muscles to their best advantage under the bright stage lights, which is why we all do it.

Many contestants find that, as they lose most of their body fat to become lean for the show, they also lose fullness in their chest. Gel inserts are common in most posing suit tops and it's not uncommon for women competing at the professional level to get breast implants. I was ahead of the pack in the fake boobs department – mine are completely plastic and looked great in the posing suit!

Finally, the competition day make-up application was an event in itself. Many of us paid the professional make-up artist to apply our game-day faces, including the false eyelashes. Others toted their entire beauty consoles with them, including mirrors and lights, to the backstage area of the contest. Contestants were roaming the halls in hot rollers and bathrobes over their suits as they sorted through the ten different pairs of earrings they brought along to make sure they had just the *right pair* to go with their hair and suits under the stage lights. Truly, this was a beauty pageant with all of its trappings and excesses.

THE JOY OF COMPETITION DAY

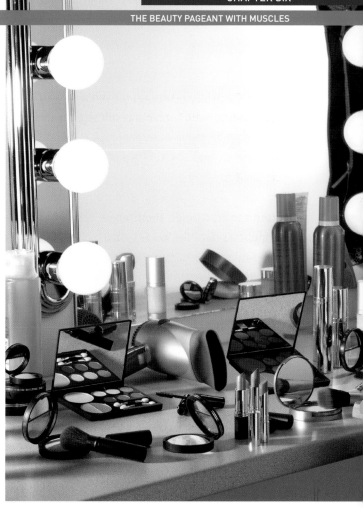

I woke up early on competition day, more excited than nervous and finding it hard to believe that the day I had been working toward for so long was finally here! I felt great, too, thanks to a very sound and healthy diet I followed during the previous week. (I avoided the dehydration and starvation plans that some competitors follow in the days prior to a show.) I was leaner than I had been in 25 years, and I looked good and had plenty of energy for the demands of the day.

It was a long day, starting with my professional make-up application at 8:30 a.m. and ending with my stage walk at 7 p.m. The segment of the day when the judges evaluated contestants started at 11 a.m. and continued until 3 p.m. We had a two-hour break until the evening show, when each contestant performed a solo stage walk and trophies were awarded, and I opted to stay at the facility during the break. I couldn't put on clothes without messing up my spray tan, so I spent that time relaxing with the other contestants and my friends who had come to cheer me on.

Despite the 10-hour duration, the events of the day flew by and my excitement and anticipation for each part of the contest carried me through it. I had signed up to compete in two different classes – one for first-time competitors and one for those age 45 and older. The staff backstage called for each class one at a time, according to a schedule, and we assembled a few minutes prior to presenting ourselves onstage. Most of us did a brief "pump up" with light weights so that our muscles looked fuller, and then we walked out as a group, standing in line across the stage. One of the judges called out the poses, and we held the pose until we were directed to change position. The lights were blinding, we were nervous and the tension was palpable. This was the test of how well each of us had prepared for posing and where practice really paid off. Less-prepared contestants would lose their ability to hold the poses under the pressure of being on stage because they lacked the stamina that comes from lots of practice. I felt well-prepared and was glad that I had practiced enough to make posing part of my muscle memory, so that my body did the right things even as my brain was overwhelmed with the pressure of being on stage.

An unexpected pleasure I found on competition day was how much fun it was to meet and get to know the other contestants. The day was like a marathon, with short bursts of intense activity on stage embedded in long stretches of waiting for the next event. A natural camaraderie formed among all of the contestants (including the men), and I was surprised at how well I came to know some of them. And forget about the stereotype of the "muscle-head" bodybuilder! Among my fellow competitors, I met a sociology professor celebrating his 60th birthday, a dentist, and the stage manager of a national news show. One of my own students was in the men's division of the show, and it was great to share this experience with him. On the whole, people were friendly, positive and encouraging. In the year since the show, I've maintained contact with several people I met and enjoy our Facebook friendships.

The last event of the day was the evening stage performance, where each contestant was formally introduced by an emcee and performed a 90-second stage walk to music. My husband, sons and a few friends came to this portion of the event, and it was during my stage walk that I felt the significance of what I had done that day. The stage walk symbolized my victory over cancer and the

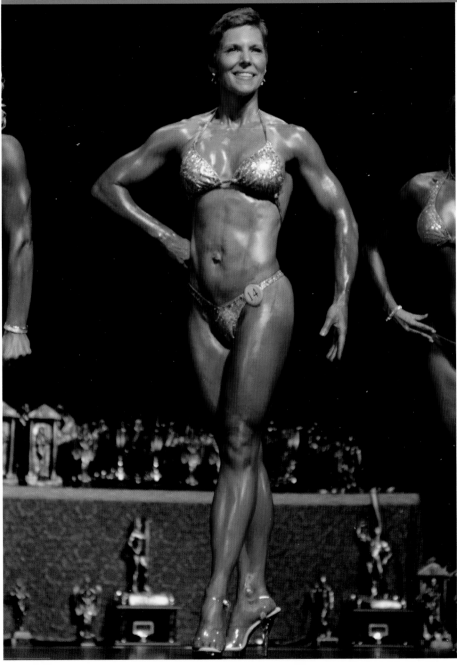

culmination of all I had worked toward since hearing my initial diagnosis. I came off of the stage and cried to the baffled, but kind, contestants and staff waiting in the wings that I felt like a winner at that moment and that it had nothing to do with whether or not I would get a trophy.

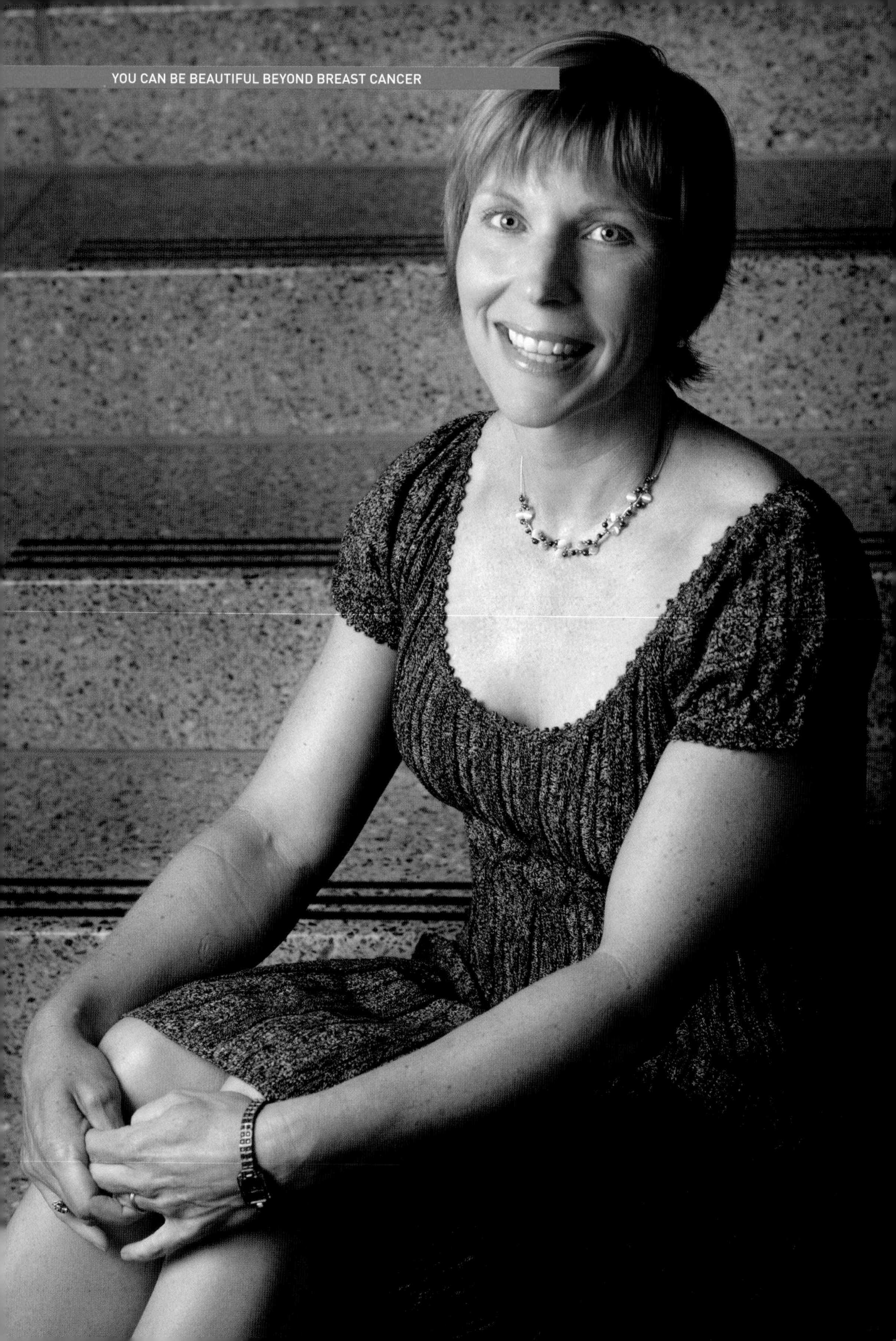

Dr. Prochaska and his colleagues have written an excellent, user-friendly book called *Changing for Good: A Revolutionary Six-Stage Program for Overcoming Bad Habits and Moving Your Life Positively Forward* (Avon Books, 1994) if you are interested in more in-depth reading on how to successfully change a habit. It provides a research-based approach to change in a format that's easy to read and apply to your life, with activities and worksheets to help you move toward your goal. It's my favorite among the self-help books for lifestyle change.

for it and collaborate with them. We get excited, and this excitement sustains us through the difficult work of making the change.

How do you arouse this emotional energy? You might read an inspirational story about someone who overcame adversity to succeed at something. Another strategy you might try is to create visual images that motivate you to want to change. An example of this is making a collage of images and phrases that inspire you and posting it where you'll see it often. You might also consider participating in a worthy cause, such as a walk to raise money for cancer research, to make your reasons for exercise more meaningful. Joining a club or class where you'll meet like-minded people with whom you can share this new passion is another great way to build your emotional investment in your new lifestyle.

Insight Three:
Weigh the benefits and the costs

Change always comes at a cost. If it didn't cost you something to change a bad habit, you would have already made the change. Don't make the mistake of telling yourself that there's nothing to like about the bad habit, because it's not true. You may find great comfort and reward at the end of a hard day by eating your favorite sweets and snacks in front of the television. Pretending that this isn't important does nothing to help you overcome it. Rather, it helps to make an honest and complete list of all the things you like about the current bad habit that you have. Allow yourself to feel how much you'll miss this bad habit and the good feelings it has given you. Then make a list of all the things you think you'll like about the new, good habits you plan to adopt. Again, put your heart into it as you imagine the many benefits that will come from your new lifestyle. You might want to do some reading or internet searching to learn more about these new habits so you can add to your list of potential benefits. Over time, the benefits of changing will become stronger and more important to you than the benefits you get from the current bad habit. It's at this point, and not until you reach this point, that you'll be ready to make the change. Instead of pushing yourself to make the habit change before you are ready, invest your time in building your list of reasons for changing to the new habit.

people to help me and a new perspective on my problems that I could not have developed on my own. There's a discernment to know when to say "yes" and when to say "no"; to know which goals are worth reaching, which ones need to change a little, and which ones need to be ditched with a sigh of relief. In the driven mode, I strain to control everything. In the called mode, I'm more flexible because I'm more trusting. It's a much kinder and gentler place from which to live my life, and now that I'm a cancer survivor, I really need kind and gentle places.

What's really amazing is that I am *more* effective, not less, when I am doing the things I feel called to do rather than the ones I feel driven to do. I'm still figuring out why, exactly, but I think it has something to do with feeling less stress, sleeping more soundly and generally being happier. It also has to do with having the peace of knowing that I'm doing what matters most and what I am meant to do. This is such a hard lesson for me to learn, though. I constantly find myself in driven mode and have to surrender it on a daily basis. One area I've struggled with this is in my training and preparation for figure competitions (I am preparing for my second competition as I write this). It's easy for training and following the diet to become a burden and feel like nothing more than work. When that happens, it's a signal to me that I need to reconsider my expectations of myself and why I'm training and competing in the first place. While trophies are wonderful, for me it has never been about winning a trophy. I compete to feel victory over cancer and to invite other cancer survivors to do the same by reaching their own goals. So when training feels like nothing but a burden, I take a few days and do it differently. I ask myself "what would feel good to do today?" Sometimes, it's a hike in the woods or some cross-country skiing if it's just snowed. When the diet feels like a burden, I treat myself to a food that's not part of my usual fare, but that I would really enjoy eating, such as a homemade cookie or fresh bread. Then I get back into the groove of feeling called to the training and diet plan because I am reminded of how much I care about my goal of competing and how much I like how I feel and look with a strong, fit body, and it becomes something I want to do again.

26 Likewise the Spirit helps us in our weakness; for we do not know how to pray as we ought, but that very Spirit intercedes k with sighs too deep for words. 27 And God, l who searches the heart, knows what is the mind of the Spirit, because the Spirit m intercedes for the saints according to the will of God. n 28 We know that all things work together for good o for those who love God, p who are called according to his purpose. 29 For those whom he foreknew he also

g Aramaic for Father   h Or 15 a spirit of

i Or by   j Other and

k Gk brothers   i Or by

l The Spirit itself bears witness   i Gk the one

m Gk he or it

n God makes all things work together fo

authorities read God makes

q Or Is it Christ Jesus :

among many brothers   8.15 Mk 14.36; Gal 4.6.   8.

POSTSCRIPT

Courage is being afraid and doing it anyway

POSTSCRIPT

Courage is being afraid and doing it anyway

In case you're wondering, I came in toward the bottom in the figure competition. I entered two categories – debut (for first-timers) and over 45 (for old-timers!) – and I came in seventh out of ten in the former and sixth out of eight in the latter. What's interesting about this is that two months before the competition, I began feeling a lot of insecurity and fear about entering it. One of my fears was that I would fall off my shoes, which didn't happen, and the other was that I would earn a low score and come in at or near the bottom. What was I thinking, putting myself on a public stage to have my post-cancer body compared to other women who had been training much longer than I had and possessed much better physiques than mine? Did I really need to do this? I spent a few sleepless nights wrestling with this fear before I could make peace with it.

I had a similar experience after I decided that I was serious about writing this book. Just like I had no experience as a competitive figure contestant, I am a novice to the world of writing and publishing books. Again, I struggled with fear that I was taking on something too big and too unfamiliar. What if no one wanted to publish or read my book? Why did I need to set myself up for rejection like that?

In both cases, I needed a reason for doing it that was bigger than my fear. It took a while, but I finally figured out what that reason is. It's all about preparing for a good death. Before you write me off as being depressing and morbid, let me explain what I mean. I once read that the purpose of life is to be ready for death when it comes. In large part, it's about creating your legacy. How will you be remembered? What impact will you have had on your family and community? Who will be better off because you lived the way you did? Entering the competition and then writing a book about it shaped my legacy as a person with courage, which simply means being scared by something but doing it anyway. You never grow unless you stretch yourself and try something new. You'll never be courageous if you don't try something scary, just like you'll never be strong if you don't pick up a heavier weight. Continuing to do the same things you've always done and

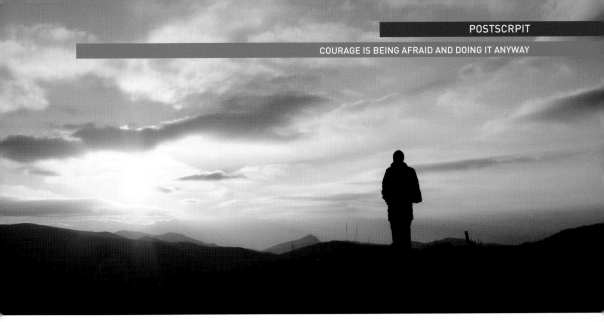

are good at does not build courage or character. You need to take a risk and try something new for that to happen.

We all die someday and, if you've survived cancer, you know your day may come sooner than you've anticipated. You realize that you don't have forever to shape your legacy; you have today.

As a mother, a college professor and the wife of a Presbyterian minister, I've devoted my life to teaching, mentoring and encouraging others. It's what I'm best at, what I was born to do and where I find the most joy in life. Ten years from now, none of my class lectures or Sunday school lessons will be remembered. What my students, our church members and my sons will remember will be my actions and attitudes around one of the most important events of my life.

There's a verse in the Bible that says "All things work together for good for those who love God and are called according to God's purpose." I've known that verse much of my life, but it's only recently that I have understood it more deeply and through experience. When I am living the life I am called to live and staying true to my priorities and values, then the pieces of my life fit together in a way that makes sense and gives me hope. It's not a quick, simple or easy realization, but it makes all of life, the good and the bad, worthwhile.

With this thought in mind, I encourage you to take heart, pursue your dream and build your legacy even as you navigate your cancer journey.

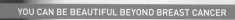

APPENDIX

The conditioning and flexibility program

APPENDIX

The conditioning and flexibility program

There are plenty of books on the market that feature resistance training programs, and some of them are actually good. Domenick and I have **not** attempted to create a general resistance training program for you after you have completed your treatment, are reasonably fit, and are ready for life beyond cancer.

We recommend the *New Rules of Lifting* series by Lou Schuler. His approach is well conceived, offering the right blend of evidence-based training programs that are challenging, effective and sound.

For those readers who are interested in training for a figure competition, our advice is to find a certified trainer who has specific experience training women for figure competitions and hire him or her to train you. The best trainers will have at least a bachelor's degree in exercise science and a personal training certification, preferably from the National Strength and Conditioning Association, National Academy of Sports Medicine, or the American College of Sports Medicine. You should also seek a trainer who has experience working with women who have gone through breast cancer treatment, if possible.

Our goal in this appendix is to provide you with muscle strengthening and flexibility exercises to help you transition through the six weeks after surgery, the cycles in between chemotherapy treatments, and throughout radiation treatments. We address the unique challenges you may face during this time, including the prevention and/or minimization of lymphedema, restoring range of motion in your shoulders, back and chest, preventing future rotator cuff injuries, and assessing your energy level and matching the training session to meet it. We have selected these exercises in particular because they are the foundation of some of the activities of daily living that you do with your upper body; in other words, doing these exercises consistently will prepare you to do all of the other activities in life that matter to you

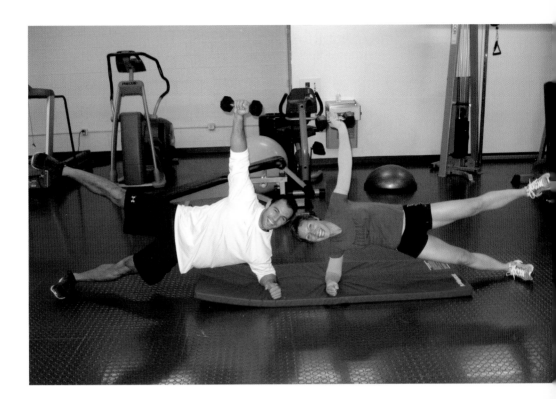

THE EXERCISES

The shoulder motions we address in the following exercises and stretches focus on increasing range of motion, flexibility and strength of the shoulder girdle region of your upper body. We focus here because the shoulder girdle (i.e., the region including your shoulders, upper back and chest) is the area most affected by your surgery. For each exercise below, Domenick and I demonstrate how to do the exercise and give you written instructions to guide you.

You can either start with no weight, just performing the motion itself, or with a level of weights or band resistance that allows you to complete the exercise at the minimum recommended repetitions with a moderate level of intensity. Once you can comfortably complete the exercises at the maximum level, it's time to increase your weight or band resistance.

Please put on your compression sleeves and hand gauntlets before you begin!

Internal Shoulder Rotation

This exercise can be performed with a partner or individually. To do the exercise on your own, you can tie the exercise band to a doorknob.

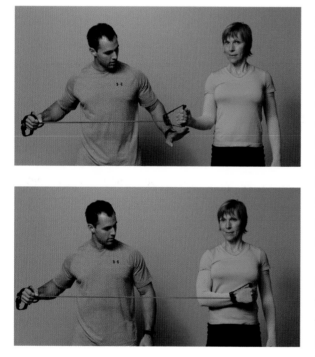

Begin with your elbow in close to your side and your working arm (the one holding the band) in an L shape as shown. Try and touch your shoulder blades together, keep them even and try and hold this position during the exercise. You start with your shoulder rotated out away from your body.

Rotate your shoulder so that your arm moves into your torso. There should be enough tension in the band to make you work, but not so much tension that you are unable to keep your elbow in at your side. You should feel the effort in your shoulder more than in your arm. You should try to keep your wrist straight during the exercise. Each repetition should take about four seconds to complete, with two seconds to move the resistance and two seconds to return to the starting position.

Release your arm and rotate your shoulder back out. Repeat this exercise with a weight that you can use 8 to 12 times with one arm and then with the other arm.

External Shoulder Rotation

This exercise is the reverse of Internal Shoulder Rotation. This exercise can be performed with a partner or individually. To do the exercise on your own you can tie the exercise band to a doorknob.

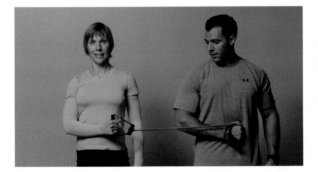

Begin with your elbow in at your side and your arm in an L shape. Your starting position is with your arm in close to your torso.

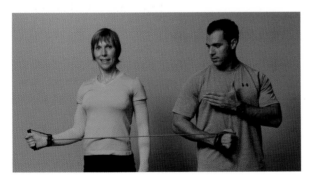

You then rotate your shoulder out, moving your arm out and the band away from your body. Let your shoulder do the work, not your arm or hand. Use enough tension to feel the work in your shoulder without moving your elbow away from your side. It's also important to keep your wrist straight on this exercise as well. Repeat with a weight that you can use 8 to 12 times with one arm, then the other.

Shoulder Elevation

You can do this exercise with or without hand weights, depending on your level of strength.

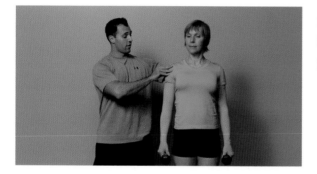

Begin with your shoulders back, even, and in a neutral position.

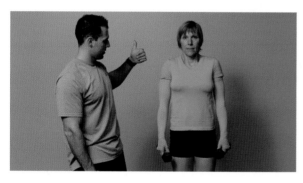

Shrug your shoulders up ...

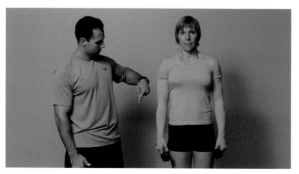

... then press them down.

Repeat with a weight that you can use 8 to 12 times.

Shoulder Depression

This is the opposite of elevation, and you use your body weight for resistance. You'll need a sturdy chair on a non-slippery surface.

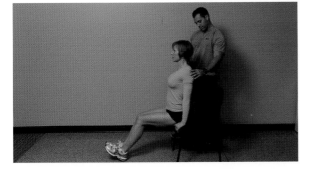

Begin by trying to touch your shoulder blades together.

Keep your shoulders even and in a neutral position and your bottom perched on the edge of the chair.

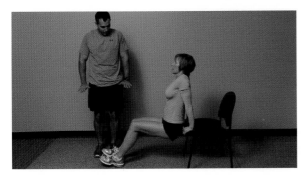

Slide your bottom forward so that it isn't on the chair and lower your body so that your shoulders are raised. It's important that you keep your arms straight and let your shoulders, not your arms, do the work.

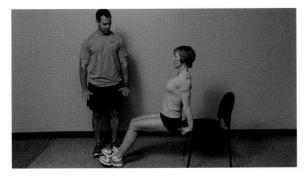

Press up, using your shoulders and not your arms, as high as you can without losing your good form and straight arms. Repeat with a weight that you can use 8 to 12 times.

Upward and Downward Shoulder Rotation

In this exercise series, you move your arms to five different points to experience both upward and downward shoulder rotation. This is a case where the five photos in sequence will probably be more instructive than the written directions, but we'll give you some anyway! You can use hand weights or not, depending on your strength level.

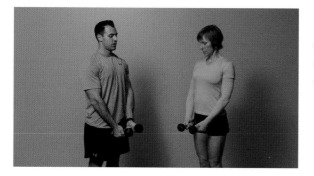

Begin with your arms down, palms in and facing each other in front of your torso.

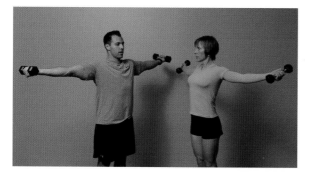

Raise your arms out to your side, turning your palms to face up.

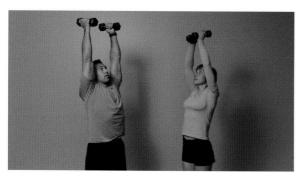

Continue raising your arms above your head, allowing your palms to face in and toward each other.

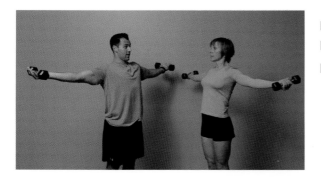

Keeping your arms straight, lower them halfway down, palms facing up.

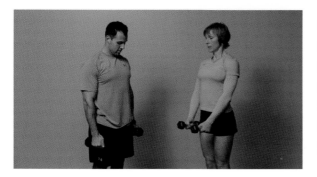

Continue to lower your straight arms so that you are back to the starting position, palms facing in. Remember, your shoulders are doing the work, not your arms.

Repeat this exercise with a weight that you can use 8-12 times.

Five Point Band Pull Apart

In this series of stretches, you'll hold a band with one end in each hand. Wrap the band around each hand so that it is tense when you pull it apart. Make it tense enough that you feel your muscles working when you pull it apart fully, but not so tense that you cannot extend your arms complete out to the side.

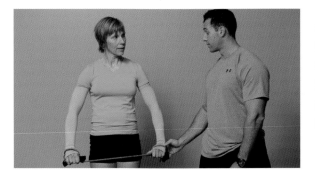

At each point, you will pull the band apart and then bring it back in. Use a slow and controlled movement at a steady pace throughout the exercise.

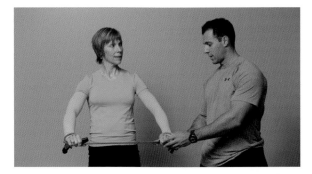

Aim to keep your arms straight so that you feel the movement in your shoulders and back.

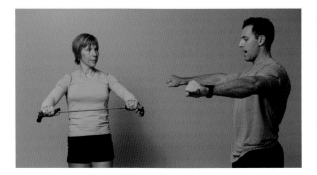

You should not be bending at the elbow as you complete this exercise. We show you the range of motion for point three and just the starting place for the other points.

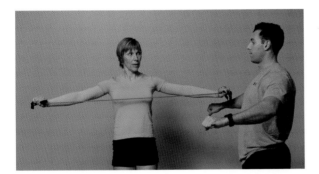

At all five points, you will start with your arms in close together, slowly pull the band apart, and then bring your arms back in. Complete 5 repetitions at each point.

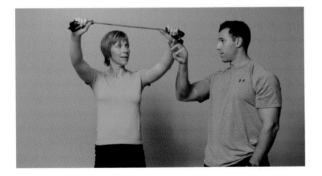

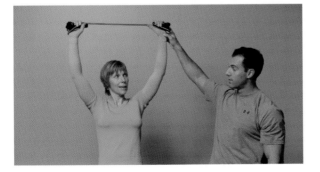

Isometric Shoulder Strengthening with a Resistance Band

In this three-point stretch, you will use a shorter band. Instead of holding handles, you want to place your hands inside the band loop and press out with the back of your hand against the band. Remember to let your shoulders do the work, not your hands. You can tie a longer band into a small loop if you don't have a short band loop. At each of the three points, you want to press out to the side, and then return your hands to the start position.

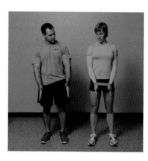 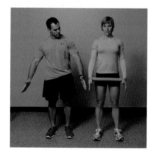

For point 1, you are standing straight with your arms down in front of you.

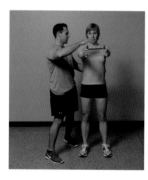 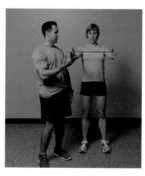

At point 2, your arms are straight and raised level with your shoulders.

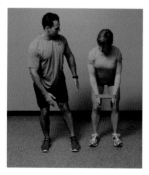 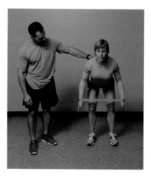

For point 3, bend your knees slightly and bend forward, keeping your head up and your back straight as you press the band.

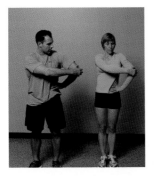

"Chicken Wing" Stretch

Place your hand on your waist, elbow out.

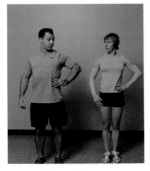

Keeping your shoulder back, reach with your opposite hand to gently hold your elbow and stretch forward.

You'll feel this stretch in your upper back around your shoulder. Stretch each side twice, holding for 15 to 30 seconds. Don't force the stretch, but relax into it as you hold it.

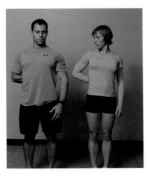

External Rotator Stretch

Place your hand behind your back, elbow out.

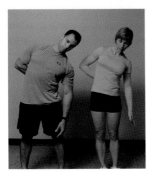

Keeping your shoulders back and even, reach down to the ground with the opposite hand. Stretch each side twice, holding for 15 to 30 seconds. Don't force the stretch, but relax into it as you hold it.

Home equipment we recommend. I do much of my training at home, and there are many pieces of useful home exercise equipment. Domenick and I particularly like and recommend the following if you are going to train at home:

THE ESSENTIAL EQUIPMENT

1. A series of pairs of Power Blocks, dumbbells and/or kettlebells, ranging from 5 to 20 pounds (or more, if you are able to work with heavier weights at this point; this recommendation is for beginners). I have both dumbbells and kettlebells, and I use them interchangeably. It's a financial investment to purchase these, and you'll need to buy more as you progress to heavier weights, but they last forever and are a staple of a home training program.

2. A stability ball. I use mine as a substitute for a bench when doing any exercise that requires me to sit, lie back or face forward. I also find it useful when working the core muscles in my torso and back.

3. Exercise bands. The beauty of exercise bands is that they are inexpensive, easy to pack and store, and can be used very effectively to increase strength, flexibility, and range of motion.

EXTRA EQUIPMENT TO ADD
VARIETY AND OPTIONS TO YOUR TRAINING

4. A step bench. I use the bench for a variety of exercises, including those for the quadriceps and hamstrings.

5. Plate Mates. These are 1.25 pound weights with magnets on them that adhere to any metal weight you are lifting. They are a great way to increase the amount of weight you are using by a small increment, which is often all I can do. Dumbbells increase in increments of 5 pounds, which is often too much of an increase for me in one step.

6.   The TRX suspension trainer. This is also a bit of an investment and requires the mounting of a hook in your ceiling, but you can connect it to almost anything outside that is stable, such as the gym equipment at your local park or a sturdy tree. I have found it to be well worth the cost. The TRX is completely portable; I did a training session on a small island off the coast of Maine while on a day-long boat excursion with my family once! I hooked the TRX up to a tree limb and did a full-body training session. The TRX adds a lot of variety and options to your home training session, allowing you to replicate gym exercises that you can't do with dumbbells or tubing.

How do I know if I am working hard enough? This is an important question, especially if you are new to weight training. It took me several months of training before I felt that I had a good sense of the right challenge level for my training sessions. Many professional trainers and fitness writers have observed that men tend to overestimate how much weight they can lift, whereas women tend to underestimate this amount. Domenick has observed that men are more likely to use poor form and body mechanics in order to lift a heavier weight, but women rarely sacrifice good form for any reason. Chances are that you will underestimate how much weight you can safely and effectively use in training until you become more confident with it, although when weight training after breast cancer treatment you want to take extra care to increase your resistance slowly and safely.

Most weight training programs will include the number of **repetitions** to complete at a time and the number of times you should perform the exercise for the specified repetitions. This is called a **set**. For example, if the program recommends that you perform three sets of squats with eight repetitions in each set, this means that you will perform eight squats, rest, do eight more squats, rest, and then do eight squats one last time. You've done three sets of eight squats.

How much weight should you be using at the start of your weight training routine? You may want to begin with no added weight at all as you learn the exercises. Once you can do them comfortably, you may want to hold a 1-5 pound weight in each hand. Start by performing 10 to 15 repetitions of the exercise, with a 60-second rest in between each complete set of repetitions. Choose a weight that allows you to work within this range. Staying within this repetition range will help you build muscle endurance, which is important for daily activities, and prepare your body for more intense exercise. It takes about 8 to 12 weeks of regular exercise, three to five days each week, to build a good base and increase muscle endurance. After 8 to 12 weeks of consistent weight training, you can reduce the number of repetitions you perform to 8-12 and slightly increase the amount of weight you are using. This will help you build more muscle mass and strength.

You should feel the need to recover during your rest periods. If you don't feel challenged, then you probably can do the exercise with a slightly heavier weight next time. If you find that in five or fewer repetitions of the exercise you are exhausted and cannot do any more repetitions, then you need to decrease the amount of weight you are using so that you can do the exercise at least 8 times.

When I first began weight training, it bothered me to have a rest period in between each set. It felt like wasted time. I was used to cardiovascular workouts, in which I was constantly moving and working for the duration of the session. I tried filling the rest period with exercise for another body part and/or stretching. Neither was a good idea and, frankly, now that I have learned what it means to lift the heaviest weights I can handle, I need the rest period to mentally regroup and catch my breath before doing the next set.

PICTURE CREDITS

+ Craig Terry   book cover, jacket-flap (2), 12, 30, 114, 129, 130 (2), 131 (2), 132 (3), 133 (3), 134 (3), 135 (2), 136 (3), 137 (3), 138 (6), 139 (4)
+ photodisc/photodisc/Thinkstock   8
+ Leslie Spencer   17, 21, 35, 36, 91, 104, 113, 118
+ Medioimages/Photodisc/Thinkstock   19
+ iStockphoto/Thinkstock   15, 20, 22, 33, 34, 39, 42, 46, 48, 60, 63, 67, 70, 72, 73, 81, 84, 88, 92, 100, 109, 111
+ Photodisc/David De Lossy/Thinkstock   24
+ Polka Dot Images/Thinkstock   25
+ Hemera/Thinkstock   16, 28, 55, 76, 99, 122, 125
+ Pixland/Jupiterimages/Thinkstock   31
+ Photos.com/Jupiterimages/Thinkstock   44
+ Digital Vision/Thinkstock   45
+ Brand X Pictures/Thinkstock   47
+ Goodshoot/Jupiterimages/Thinkstock   50
+ Photodisc/Andy Sotiriou/Thinkstock   68
+ Photodisc/Thinkstock   78
+ Creatas/Thinkstock   79
+ Stockbyte/John Foxx/Thinkstock   95
+ Comstock/Jupiterimages/Thinkstock   96
+ Comstock/Thinkstock   107
+ Stockbyte/Thinkstock   126

Cover Design: Sabine Groten
Cover Graphic: Hemera/Thinkstock